$\mathscr{F}$INDING $\mathscr{K}$ATE

The Unlikely Journey of 20th Century Healthcare Advocate Kate Macy Ladd

Meryl Carmel

Open Door Publications

Finding Kate
The Unlikely Story of 20th Century Healthcare
Advocate Kate Macy Ladd
Copyright© 2018 by Meryl Carmel

ISBN: 978-0-9981208-8-1

Published by
Open Door Publications
2113 Stackhouse Dr.
Yardley, PA 19067
www.OpenDoorPublications.com

Cover design: Eric Labacz, www.labaczdesign.com
Front cover photo: Kate and Comus at Sunnybranch Farm, circa 1910
(Courtesy of Edith Macy Shoenborn)

For Doug, my North Star and companion on every journey.

"Free to choose a life of ease and pleasure she has been guided since childhood by a consuming desire to be of service to those in suffering or need or eager for education and growth. A self denying champion of the good and fair in life she has added to her many other deeds of generosity also the sponsorship of science and its contributions to the welfare of mankind..."

From the Josiah Macy Jr. Foundation Archives
New York, New York

Preface

WHY WAS I SO DRAWN TO KATE MACY LADD? Looking back, it appears that our lives were meant to intersect. Once I decided to find Kate, I had to dig below the surface to understand who she was and why she responded to people in need of care and compassion. Uncannily, as I searched for her motivations, I illuminated my own. Bringing to light aspects of another woman's life is a way of showing respect for her unrecognized contributions, and I had been training for a mission of this kind since I was a little girl. I have long yearned to tell another woman's story. At an early age I was inspired to learn about people from the past when I first discovered the *Patriot Signature Biography* series at the library. For me, these tales brought to life the prominent Americans who explored the continent and established the nation, including a lone female, Elizabeth Griscom Betsy Ross (aka Elizabeth Calhoun).

In 1960, the story of Betsy Ross particularly captivated me because it was the first biography of a woman that I ever read. My teachers offered scant information about the achievements of women. Betsy was the exception. I learned that she was born into a Quaker family, married three times, and became the mother of many daughters. Her defining achievement was the creation of the first American flag. I accepted that while the "great men" explored new lands, waged war, and led the nation, this seamstress lived simply in my hometown of Philadelphia. I embraced the private and domestic nature of her contribution to history, and I was motivated to pick up needle and thread and attempt to sew a small sampler in her honor. I eagerly visited her home, and it was there, in the tiny row house on Arch Street, that history came to life for me for the first time.

For years thereafter I believed, as I had been taught, that at the invitation of George Washington, my female heroine spun the thread, wove the cloth, and sewed the first American flag. Never mind that the legend of Betsy Ross was just that—a fabrication. Over time, I

was astounded to learn that much of what I had read in my history
books was inaccurate and that key information about women's lives
and contributions to American society was limited or missing
altogether.

For a time, I was enamored with the field of archeology,
delicately unearthing the remnants of long-ago lives with small hand
tools and determination. In graduate school I gravitated to the study of
Colonial women and the twentieth century historians who were
committed to illuminating women's lives through a careful
reconstruction of the past. Happily, I discovered the work of one
Colonial woman who was a historian in her own right: Mercy Otis
Warren. A member of an eminent New England family, this
remarkable woman wrote an early and comprehensive account of the
Revolutionary War published in 1805. In three volumes, and more
than 1,300 pages, her *History of the Rise, Progress, and Termination
of the American Revolution* was praised by political leaders of the
day. President Thomas Jefferson was so impressed with Warren's
insightful work that he presented copies of the book to all of his
cabinet members.

My own research focused on Colonial era Quaker women who
lived in Maryland and Delaware at roughly the same time that Betsy
Ross lived in Philadelphia. Through an analysis of primary sources, I
reconstructed the stories of their lives, seeking to provide fresh
insights about women of the period. The female Friends I studied
were generous spirits who tended hearth and home and, like Betsy,
spun thread to weave into cloth to sew garments for their families. In
the latter half of the eighteenth century, however, despite their
inherently domestic roles, the Quaker women I came to know
assumed decidedly public roles traveling from their farms to local
court houses to sign and witness the deeds of manumission that
legally freed their slaves from servitude. It was humbling to document
and contemplate the participation of conscientious women setting
aside their household duties to participate in their society's effort to
eliminate slaveholding by 1792. My experience documenting the
actions of rural Quaker women only confirmed for me the need to
research and retrieve history about women's lives. Ideally, I hoped to
find one woman to be the subject of my future work. She would be
generous of spirit and, like my female Friends, a person who showed

compassion toward others. I was not sure just how I would find her.

It was not until 2007 when I realized that my subject had been waiting for me in the shadows a short way from my home. Her name was Kate Macy Ladd, and as I read in the park brochure about the women's convalescent home she established right on her estate, I knew that this was an act that set her apart from other women of her era, and that it represented Kate's extraordinary compassion toward women. I was sure that it was the key to understanding her, and that I must dutifully bring it to light. *Finding Kate* is her story, and in a way my own.

How the Journey Began

I<small>T ALL STARTED WITH A HIKE IN EARLY FALL</small> 2007. On that September Sunday, I set out for a local county park I had not visited before. The colors of autumn lacked confidence, and a sunless sky muted them even further. Yet, vast verdant lawns extended in every direction. Overlooking it all sat an imposing mansion, the jewel in one of the region's foremost grand estates: Natirar. The name conveys a hint of opulence entirely in keeping with the considerable cachet of the area; but significantly, the property's southern edge is defined by a narrow bubbling river, a branch of the Raritan, and although it diminishes the mystique of an exotic name, Natirar is merely an anagram for Raritan.

The lush and expansive area between Morristown and Somerville, New Jersey, became host to a great variety of country homes or "cottages" in the Gilded Age, resulting in an elegant estate enclave that continued to expand well into the twentieth century. Affluent industrialists and their families populated Natirar's neighbor estates. More recently, Natirar itself has been the home of the King of Morocco, an intimate of the rich and famous. Malcolm Forbes and Jackie Kennedy Onassis were among the elite who called these hills home at one time or another. As I scanned the landscape, I recalled that President Dwight D. Eisenhower used to fish the very river within my gaze.

Connected to New York by rail, the Somerset Hills made an idyllic residence for those with city business ties and cultural interests, but who wished to come home to a "country" retreat. It was easy to succumb to the allure of the Somerset Hills, originally known as the Upper Raritan Valley of New Jersey. The area is tucked away in a peaceful and picturesque corner of the Garden State. Since the mid-nineteenth century wealthy individuals had been discovering the distinct pleasures of summering just forty miles west of New York City; before the close of the century, many chose to become part of the more permanent colony that was developing in these gentle and luxurious hills.

On that autumn day in 2007, as I completed the pleasant loop trail, I noticed a park kiosk with a wooden box labeled "Trail Maps." Inside was a well-designed publication, *Welcome to Natirar,* which provided more than the promised map. I learned that Natirar is a 411-acre property located in Somerset County, divided among the municipalities of Peapack-Gladstone (247 acres), Far Hills (124 acres), and Bedminster (40 acres). The North Branch of the Raritan River and the Peapack Brook traverse the property. Most importantly, I discovered that Natirar was formerly the estate of Kate Macy Ladd and Walter Graeme Ladd. The property features extensive lawns and woodlands, river access, and scenic views as well as historic farm buildings and various other residential structures and outbuildings dating from the mid-eighteenth through mid-nineteenth centuries. As the brochure notes, "Natirar presents a unique opportunity for a single property to preserve, showcase, and interpret many aspects of the area's rich architectural, cultural, historic, and archeological heritage."

But I was more interested in the people of Natirar. Catherine ("Kate") Everit Macy Ladd and her husband, Walter Graeme Ladd, began to acquire land in Somerset County in April 1905. Eventually, they created one of the largest estates in the area, Natirar, encompassing some thousand acres stretching from what is now Route 206 on the west, across the North Branch of the Raritan River on the east, and from Highland Avenue in Peapack on the north, to what is now Route 202 on the south. The Ladd's brick, 40-room Tudor-style mansion was completed in 1912. It was designed by Guy Lowell, a Boston-born architect who is most famous for his design of the Boston Museum of Fine Arts and the New York County Court House on Foley Square in Manhattan.

The Ladds and their wealth fascinated me, but it was a brief paragraph in the park brochure that riveted my attention and brought together the "perfect storm" of personal and professional interests that led to this book. I read that in 1908 Mrs. Ladd established a convalescent facility on the Natirar estate, originally at "Maple Cottage," a large residence that once stood along Peapack Road where "deserving gentlewomen who are compelled to depend upon their own exertions for support shall be entertained without charge, for periods of time while convalescing from illness, recuperating from impaired health, or otherwise in need of rest."

The fact that the estate's original owner, Kate Macy Ladd chose to provide a convalescent home on this stunning property for women "who are compelled to depend upon their own exertions for support" stopped me in my tracks. I am well aware that in the nineteenth and twentieth centuries, as today, the activities of wealthy women included entertaining; attending luncheons, dinners, and society parties; supporting the opera and theater; and participating in garden clubs and literary societies and, as time permitted, doing their bit for those less fortunate. But the notion of an affluent woman, more than a century ago, establishing a women's convalescent facility on her property struck me as remarkable and unique.

I left the park that day feeling intrigued, excited, and certain that I must know more about Natirar and Kate. I was simply following my curiosity at first. Of course, that is how all good journeys begin. I love to explore the physical world, navigating trails with the assurance of compass and map; but as an amateur archeologist and historian I have been trained to navigate through time—to sift through earth, sand, shells, paper, and myriad fragments of the past. Whether hiking the present or sifting the past, I have learned that following a trail requires persistence and faith and, as my search for Kate has taught me, a willingness to accept that the story of another woman's life falling into my hands, piece by piece, through amazing coincidences and connections neither of us could have imagined, could bring with it an obligation to tell her story.

A stroke of luck further convinced me to follow Kate's trail. Just when I was ready to give up, source material being scarce, I stumbled upon a memoir written by her in 1929. It was offered online by an antiquarian bookseller in the Adirondacks. The bookseller's tasteful website provided a telephone contact number. I decided to call and a pleasant voice answered the phone immediately. I learned that the memoir was found in a carton filled with textbooks at a home on Long Island. Within minutes, the transaction was complete. My first primary source had been purchased and shipped by day's end, and I was reminded of how much has changed since 1929. Today an online search makes it possible to hunt for almost anything in the comfort of your own home. Digging in the past can be merely a click away.

Nevertheless, I had a sense that it would require time and persistence to unravel and reconstruct Kate's past.

Kate's memoir arrived in pristine condition, 269 cream-colored pages interspersed with copies of nineteenth century photographs, carefully protected by thin sheets of tissue paper. I eagerly opened the leather cover to find a picture of six-year-old Kate, a shy-looking child, her delicate face dominated by her dark eyes. The volume is inscribed: "For dearest Helen with fond love from Kate."

When Kate began her memoir, the stock market had recently plummeted, and even though her personal wealth was not affected, she felt distressed over the misfortune of others. By the fall of 1929, she was troubled by a variety of family and household issues as well. Her husband, Walter, suggested that she write a sketch about her life. He thought this might be a distraction from her worries, and Kate took his recommendation to heart.

Her memoir spans the years 1863 to 1929. In the preface Kate attributes her joy in life to her early religious training and faith in a Higher Power, her splendid parents, devoted husband, fine and capable physicians, and her greatest blessing, "a most unusual woman whom I had as a companion for twenty-five years." With the completion of her memoir, which was published by the venerable Mosher Press in Portland, Maine, Kate felt temporarily uplifted. She was pleased when the beautifully bound books arrived at her New Jersey home, and she carefully personalized them for friends and relatives.

Further investigation reveals that a few months later, perhaps emboldened by her recent "literary" accomplishment, as well as appreciative of the preservation of her wealth, Kate shifted gears. She moved forward with a plan that had long been on her mind. Inspired by the example of generations of family involvement in charitable work, and moved by a desire to honor her beloved father, she established a medical foundation in his memory. Simply called "The Josiah Macy Jr. Foundation," it was a significant aspect of her philanthropic legacy and yet one that has remained in the shadows. Reflecting upon Kate's creation of Maple Cottage for convalescing women, and her establishment of a medical foundation that persists to this day I became more determined than ever to "find" Kate.

Chapter 1

KATE EVERIT MACY WAS BORN at 55 West Twenty-Eighth Street, New York City, at a time when a child of privilege entered the world in the privacy and comfort of home, on April 6, 1863 at 8 a.m., the Monday after Easter. It had been a snowy winter followed by a muddy early spring, and Kate arrived just as the roads were drying out and the daffodils were peeping up along country lanes. She was greeted by a family circle filled with love. Upon learning the news of her birth her mother's female relatives made their way to her bedside to visit and inspect the small bundle nestled by her breast while the men made haste to attend the St. Nicholas Society gathering at Delmonico's. Kate was the second child in the family; she and her sister Mary, not much more than a baby herself, were showered with attention.

The timing of Kate's arrival could not have been more auspicious: It raised her family's spirits immeasurably. Most Americans felt more apprehension than joy in those days. The front page of *The New York Times* carried grim news of the Civil War. Although the tide of victory appeared to be turning toward the north as the Union cavalry overwhelmed Rebel strongholds throughout Tennessee, her pacifist relatives did not celebrate. They were not buoyed by the news of Union triumph with Vicksburg under siege and Fort Sumter facing bombardment. The Macys had traded in southern cotton for years and had strong bonds with their Alabama kin; however, they were not Confederate sympathizers. They were northerners, big city merchants, and members of the Society of Friends who opposed slavery. As humanitarians, they were horrified by any kind of cruelty and suffering and outraged by accounts of the goings-on at Richmond where it was reported that desperate women raged in the streets. Hungry and equipped with clubs and stones (and according to some accounts guns) they broke into government stores to secure food and clothing for themselves and their children. The

Macys spoke out against injustice for years to come; their sympathy for unfortunate women and children never diminished.

Kate was the newest addition to the ninth generation of Macys in America. Her parents were Caroline Louise Everit, always known as Carrie, and Josiah Macy Jr. Their families had been well acquainted through the New York Friends Meeting as well as business for years. As leather manufacturers and oil merchants they had more in common than might meet the eye. The family lines intermingled as the old Quakers tended to worship, socialize, and marry within the Religious Society of Friends. As Kate's Grandfather Macy put it, a man should "look for a wife not far from the chimney of his father's house."

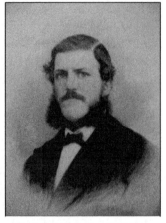

Josiah Macy Jr., 1838-1876 *(Courtesy of the Macy Family)*

Carrie and Josiah were wed on the bride's twentieth birthday, December 9, 1858, in a simple Quaker ceremony at her home, witnessed by relatives and friends who signed the marriage certificate, as was the custom. They made the round of wedding calls to family members all over the city, and soon thereafter the newlyweds traveled to Niagara Falls, Canada, with Josiah's parents, Eliza Jenkins and William Hussey Macy. At that time, Niagara Falls was considered one of the world's greatest natural wonders, recently immortalized in Frederic Edwin Church's majestic oil painting, "Niagara." The nuptial journey (as honeymoons were called) was memorialized with an early photograph of the two couples perched self-consciously on a simple wooden bench, the mighty falls cascading in the background. Boaters, swimmers, barrel riders, and tightrope walkers—all manner of thrill seekers—sought fame and fortune at the falls. The first to attempt a dangerous stunt was a showman trained in the tradition of the European circus; he walked the tightrope over the gushing waters just months after the Macy wedding trip. Even more stunning than this was the derring-do of a young woman who crossed the cavernous gorge walking backward on a taut wire. A paper bag covered her head, a wooden peach basket sheathed each foot!

The newlyweds were aware of the notoriety attached to the place of their first journey as man and wife. Although they were members of the Society of Friends, they were not provincials. With their nuptial trip to Niagara they were very much in the forefront of the customs of the time. They were stunned, however, to learn that some men and women had become fixated with Niagara for another reason, which no one mentioned within earshot of children. The eerily beautiful falls were like a magnet to would-be suicides whose desperate deeds were recorded in newspapers throughout the country, shocking even perfect strangers.

Leaving the excitement associated with Niagara behind, Carrie and Josiah settled down into a calm and predictable daily routine that was consistent with their similar upbringing. For Carrie this meant managing her first household aided by a housemaid, a task for which she had been in training for years. She aimed to perfect the creation of a home that would serve as a refuge for her husband, who went off to the offices of Josiah Macy and Sons on Front Street early each morning. They lived close to Josiah's parents, renting a variety of homes for a number of years, and were never too far from Carrie's family. The young couple regularly visited with their relations, spending Sundays at Quaker meeting, followed by tea or supper on Twenty-First Street in Manhattan or in Brooklyn Heights, a short ferry ride away.

Chapter 2

CAROLINE LOUISE EVERIT WAS THE DAUGHTER of Beulah Elma Kirby and Valentine Everit, well-respected Brooklyn Friends. The Everits were Brooklyn and Long Island people going back before the Revolutionary War. Carrie and her siblings were raised in the fashionable part of town. At the time of her birth, Brooklyn was the seventh most populated municipality in the nation, and her father was considered one of Brooklyn's elite as affirmed in a guide to Brooklyn's wealthiest citizens. As a successful leather merchant, he was a member of a circle of businessmen that included the Macys. Kate's grandfathers were well acquainted through the Leather Merchants Association and Bank of which William Macy was president, as well as their Friends Meeting.

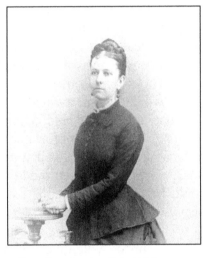

Caroline Louise Everit Macy, 1838-1898 *(Courtesy of the Macy Family)*

Valentine Everit operated a tannery in Brooklyn and conducted commerce at 32 Ferry Street in an area called "the Swamp" where the top leather manufacturers congregated. He had worked there since his youth alongside his father, Kate's great-grandfather Thomas Everit (also spelled Everett), who carried on several businesses before settling on the leather trade. Born and raised in 1764, people called Thomas Everit a scholar. He was said to be happiest when surrounded by his books, yet he was a practical man and understood the need to earn a living so he exchanged his beloved volumes of Shakespeare and Greek and Roman history for a butcher's knife and apron. He and his brother assumed their father's stall in the Old Fly Market at the foot of Maiden Lane. This was the site of slave auctions prior to becoming a well-known food market where meat, fish, and produce were hawked under covered stalls.

The Everit men had been butchers for generations without interruption until Thomas Everit's father took leave of his stall to go off to fight in the Revolutionary War. He joined the Long Island militia, and he served as second lieutenant in Captain Adolph Waldon's Light Horse Brigade, participating in the Battle of Long Island. This was the first major action of the war fought under General George Washington and a major defeat for the Americans; it resulted in their evacuation of New York in August 1776.

Lt. Everit was never a member of the Religious Society of Friends. It was not until after he married and tried his hand at farming at Hempstead that his son Thomas Everit, Jr. joined the Society of Friends in what was a thriving Quaker community that included the Titus, Hicks, Underhill, and Willets clans, with whom the family's future would be intertwined. The Society of Friends informed much of what the Everits and Macys believed and chose to do in life. Although he was comfortable following the ways of the Friends, Thomas Jr. was not so well suited for farming, and so he and his wife, Susannah Valentine, returned to Brooklyn where good land for homes could be acquired cheaply. Uniting with his brothers he became a heavy leather dealer.[1]

The leather business had its ups and downs, but eventually was passed on to Valentine, who referred to himself as a leather manufacturer. He was involved with a group of local businessmen, many of whom were Quakers. He built a store and carried on trade on Ferry Street. With improvements in production methods, Valentine engaged in a far less gruesome enterprise than did his forebears. In an earlier period, the Everits had earned their living butchering pigs and cows; while in Nantucket, the Macys slaughtered whales for their highly prized sperm oil. By the time Kate was born, both sides of the family had progressed to new trades and prospered in their businesses. As butchers, tanners, whalers, and merchants they were all hardworking men who passed down their Quaker values of modesty, philanthropy, and compassion—values that would one day define Kate as well.

While the Macys often seemed larger-than-life to Kate, she knew far less about her Everit ancestors. Her grandfather Valentine shared stories about his father's generous and charitable nature, explaining that he and fellow Brooklyn Friends were committed to aiding the sick and poor and ensuring that fuel and foodstuffs were available to those in need throughout the difficult winter months. Along with a small band of Quaker merchants Thomas Everit pledged to rid a particularly unsavory downtown district of a level of vice, filth, and poverty said to rival the notorious Five Points area of New York City. Joining together, the men managed to clean up those mean streets. While there is no record of how this was accomplished, their efforts were recognized with gratitude by residents in the vicinity and acknowledged in the press. Although they were modest people, Kate's relatives did not mind good publicity, and they also seemed to relish having their images captured by photographers who appeared to be setting up studios on every corner in Brooklyn and Manhattan. Kate's home was filled with portraits, daguerreotypes, hand-painted miniatures on ivory (sometimes encased in gemstones). Eventually, photographs—countless photographs—were grandly displayed in sterling frames or placed in elaborately decorated velvet, satin, or leather-covered books so that they might easily be viewed and admired.

Kate's dearth of information about the early Everits stemmed from the fact that her mother, Carrie, had no memory of her altruistic grandfather Thomas and so she shared little information about him or his wife, Susannah Valentine. This was in stark contrast to Kate's father, Josiah, who was more well-versed in his family story. However, Carrie's father, Valentine Everit, had a pair of sisters whom Carrie knew well. They were called Phebe and Catherine; Catherine was the first Catherine Everit, Kate was the third. Phebe was the last Phebe in the line.

The daughters of a successful merchant such as Thomas Everit, whose American roots were planted in Connecticut in 1632, could expect to marry into the family of a wealthy businessman, and Catherine Everit managed just that. At age sixteen she wed Robert Titus Hicks, the son of Whitehead Hicks, a prosperous lumber merchant and one of the founders of the Seventh Ward where the early New York merchants located their homes and businesses. He followed in his father's mercantile footsteps, establishing a chandlery business at Crane's Wharf near Fulton Market. In time he owned a fleet of sailing vessels engaged in the South American and the West Indies trade, making Catherine a very wealthy young matron. Carrie's Hicks relations retired to Poughkeepsie and built an elegant country seat, after which the Everits saw them sparingly. It was not until her husband died that Catharine Hicks returned to Brooklyn, living on Hicks Street near Everit kin.

Phebe did not fare as well. Marriage prospects for a second daughter were often somewhat dimmer; in this case her father's sudden reversal of fortune may have also worked against her. The family owned a showplace of a house on Willow Street where blue Catawba grapes ripened on vines in a sunny garden. This fine address was a gathering place for local society and enabled the Everit daughters to mingle with Brooklyn's finest families. But once the family's fortune dwindled it was necessary to sell their showplace and move into a more ordinary house. Their society-driven existence abruptly ended, and Thomas died not long thereafter. Phebe Everit was consigned to share a home with her widowed mother; after her mother died, Phebe joined Carrie's family.

Phebe's unfortunate life might have provided food for thought for her great-niece Kate. Catherine Everit had made a spectacular marriage but her younger sister was left out in the cold. Kate knew that men had greater control of their lives than women. To marry or not was their own decision; bachelors were well-thought-of while spinsters were disdained. An unattached gentleman was the beneficiary of feminine fawning and attention, sought after as an escort and included on the guest list for all the best society occasions. Everyone had such a man in the family: a charming, gracious raconteur, well-traveled and always good company. A double standard governed relations between the sexes and gave women limited options in life.

This could have been somewhat confusing to a girl raised in an egalitarian nineteenth century Quaker family. Female Friends were educated and encouraged to possess a distinct voice and develop leadership skills in their Women's Meetings. Their opinions about religious and community matters were sought and granted equal consideration. And the women of Nantucket from whom Kate descended were strong and independent by necessity.

Kate also saw the traditional Quaker influence in the way her maternal grandmother dressed. Beulah Everit, the picture of sweetness with delicate features, wore prim, dark frocks that never went out of style. Her gowns had long full skirts of wool or silk for First Day, the simple bodice enhanced only by a sheer lawn kerchief to match her cap. Over her shoulders she wore a shawl to precisely match her dress. A special occasion or a formal portrait called for greater finery but the effect was always the same. A ruffle here or there did nothing to alter the overall proper and buttoned up look.

Unlike Beulah Everit, Carrie Macy was very modern and would rebel mightily against what she considered old-time Quaker dress; she was what some called a worldly Quaker. Carrie passed on her love of fashion to Kate, who never tired of dressing up. Carrie's silks, laces, and furs were always exquisite; she never wore a prim little white cap.

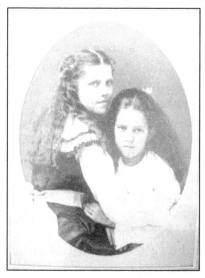

Mary "Mae" Kingsland Macy, age 10, and Kate Everit Macy, age 8 *(Courtesy of the Macy Family)*

In her youth a leghorn bonnet, or later a French Chapeau created by Vennet in Paris was more her mode, and her hair was always perfectly dressed with swirls and braids woven throughout her thick, dark tresses. When she finally traveled to Paris she kept the dressmakers busy filling trunks for the trip home with skirts and dresses and down-filled petticoats for herself and friends. She was not insistent on Worth Couture like her favorite sister-in-law Mary Kingsland, who patronized the popular high-fashion design house whenever she visited Paris. And yet in a way, she did share Mary's taste for expensive finery; Carrie was mad for old Venetian and Flemish lace. After they married, Josiah spoiled her with costly antique laces. She had exquisite pieces transformed into elaborate dress collars that made a real statement—what a contrast they were to her mother's simply adorned necklines and lawn collars! While she owned a few pieces of ancient lace, Beulah Everit's taste was more subdued. It was not for lack of money—she could have been outfitted by the finest dressmakers in New York—but this was of no interest to her. She was simply prim and modest in every way. It was her way of life.

Another Quaker custom that appealed to Kate was the simple Friends marriage ceremony even though she would not follow the custom herself. It is a hallmark of Quaker matrimony that the couple undertakes marriage on equal terms, neither one promising obedience to the other. No one said "I promise to love, honor and *obey* 'til death do us part." It was universally accepted that couples should have "no rule but love between them." Obedience was expected based on cooperation. Once vows were exchanged and the congregation observed a brief period of silence, the large marriage certificate, carefully written and embellished on fine paper, would be displayed and signed by those who witnessed the ceremony. Beulah Kirby's sister Sarah Ann and Valentine Everit's brother Henry had become man and wife following this distinctly Quaker tradition several years before Beulah's marriage, and they were among the family witnesses when Kate's grandparents were joined in matrimony.

Kate assumed that it was through their respective siblings that her shy, older grandfather, a thirty-eight-year-old bachelor, came to know and eventually court her grandmother who was a dozen years his junior. She wondered if her grandmother had fallen in love with his romantic sounding name of Valentine. It was his mother's family name, one which would appear in future male generations despite its cherubic ring. The couple married the day after St. Valentine's Day, and their first child, Carrie, arrived before year's end.

Beulah and Valentine raised a good size brood, most of which reached adulthood—no small feat in those days of high childhood mortality. Their son Thomas would become his father's partner. He married Caroline Lansing and their first baby, a son, was born soon after Kate. His death fifteen months later struck fear in the hearts of Carrie and Josiah; perhaps this explains why they tended to hover over Kate and her sister so closely. Happily, Thomas and his wife produced three girls in quick succession: Anna, Helen, and Beulah; however, the Everit line ended in that generation.

By the 1850s Beulah and Valentine Everit owned a handsome

brownstone at 64 Clark Street, a fashionable address. The Brooklyn neighborhood streets were graced with lovely names: Willow, Orange, Pineapple, and Love Lane, and lined with cherry trees whose puffy blossoms were softly scented in the spring.

During her youth, Carrie's neighborhood was a peaceful and comfortable place and boasted some of the finest homes in the vicinity. It was an elite enclave of merchants and professional men, worlds apart from the hectic and crowded wards of Manhattan. In her rarefied corner of Brooklyn Heights, Carrie Everit attended Quaker meeting and, with her mother's patient guidance, mastered the lessons of Victorian domesticity while maintaining a slightly independent bent. Always a quick study, she was tutored in reading, writing, and mathematics and she was known to have a keen head for figures. As a young lady she traveled over to Manhattan by ferry to visit friends, attend religious gatherings, or enjoy shopping along the Ladies' Mile. When she decided to marry a young man from across the East River she felt comfortable knowing it would always be easy to return home to the Heights. By the late 1850s dependable ferry service existed between Fulton Street and Lower Manhattan, with travel time under five minutes and the fare just a few cents each way.[2]

While she prepared for a life of marriage and family, her brother Thomas operated under the wing of their father, learning the tanner's trade and participating in mercantile affairs as heir apparent to the Everit leather manufacturing business. At home, Carrie, and to some extent her sister Catherine, helped with their two younger siblings, Anna, who married Laurence Hurlburt, the son of a Utica lawyer, and baby of the family Edward Augustus, who must have been a surprise to Beulah at age forty-two. Before he arrived there were two other little babes who were not long in this world, William Henry and Valentine, Jr.

The youngest Everit child, Edward, was just age four or five when Carrie wed and was more of an older brother to Kate and Mary; he was expected to keep a watchful eye out for them as they became young ladies and often accompanied them on excursions and holidays, which Carrie paid for. She was dependably generous with her less affluent siblings, bringing them along when the family traveled and making sure they enjoyed simple luxuries, and was considered a model daughter and sister: dutiful, loving, and considerate. After she died, her relatives were financially set for life.

Carrie and Josiah's marriage ceremony took place at the Everit home. The newlyweds made a striking pair. Carrie was pretty and petite, with dark hair and penetrating eyes to match. Josiah was tall, angular, and blue-eyed, with mutton chops. He was infatuated by his bride, and letters reveal that he remained so always. He believed that Carrie was a perfect wife except for the fact that unlike the Macys she was never much of a letter writer. He said that this was the only thing that she could not do equal to anyone.

Carrie Macy was passionate about many things. She was descended from people who, like the Macys, were committed to helping those less fortunate, a pledge that increased as her own fortune grew, and she instilled her values in her children. If someone needed to borrow money she rarely refused to make the loan, and never expected to be repaid. Anonymous acts of generosity were her hallmark, and this impressed Kate, who wanted to follow her mother and use her inherited wealth to "do good" in a quiet and unobtrusive manner.

Chapter 3

KATE'S FATHER JOSIAH MACY JR., THIRD SON of William H. Macy Sr. and Eliza Leggett Jenkins, grew up in New York City, residing with his parents, two sisters, and three brothers at 40 East Twenty-First Street. In the 1840s the city streets were lined with trees on both sides, leafy butternuts that gave the neighborhood a country feel. The Macy house was surrounded by a garden dotted with fruit trees and protected from the hustle and bustle of the neighborhood by a wrought iron fence on all sides. At one time, a cow or two grazed on the property—hard to imagine in the middle of New York City.

Although he spent his entire life in New York, Josiah's family was rooted in Nantucket. With the birth of his sister Mary's son Cornelius, the Macys began to significantly enlarge their presence in their adopted city. Although the enormous families produced in the Nantucket days were a thing of the past, the Macys spawned a substantial tribe of boys and girls. Engaged in business and living in close proximity, the family was no place for secrets. Everyone was quite involved in each other's lives. Kate and her cousins were great friends; they played, attended Sunday meeting, and went on holidays together. A stable and storied American family, the Macys shared their ups and downs as close families do, and Kate learned the importance of love, loyalty, and support.

Josiah's line can be traced back to the first American Macys, Thomas and Sarah from Wiltshire, Chilmark Parish, England. Their ancestral home was southwest of London where the family raised grain and livestock. Thomas Macy was a skilled weaver, but the local economy was weak. Life was particularly difficult for religious dissenters such as the Macys who were "Brethren," a branch of Christianity that became known as Baptists, and like the Puritans and others who did not recognize the Church of England, Thomas Macy faced religious persecution. An increasingly hostile environment in England spawned a "Great Migration" of English settlers to the West

Indies and Massachusetts. The possibility of religious liberty and freedom from the rigid British class system was enough to convince the newly married Thomas and Sarah Macy to leave Britain.

The Macys braved a two- or three-month transatlantic crossing, arriving in America about 1635. They settled briefly in Newbury in the Massachusetts Bay Colony and more permanently in Salisbury and began to raise a family and carve out a new life. Thomas met with some early success: He set up a saw mill (wood being a more critical commodity than a weaver's cloth) and became involved in local affairs. With the passage of time, however, he began to question the entrenched Puritan theocracy—as a Baptist he remained an outsider, in a place where Puritans received preferential treatment—moreover, they quickly forgot about the way they had been persecuted in England. According to the *Macy Genealogy* written by Kate's uncle Silvanus and published in 1868, "No sooner had the Pilgrim fathers found themselves to be free from religious oppression of their native land, than they assumed the right to dictate, and usurp the power to say which was the true church, and to condemn the unbelievers."[1]

By the latter 1650s emissaries of George Fox, who founded the Society of Friends, had reached the colonies to preach their message of the inner light of God and enjoy religious freedom. The Puritan clergy immediately branded them "witches and heretics [and] the heart-rending cruelties of the Reformation were re-enacted."[2] Peaceful Quaker men, women, and children were routinely routed out of town or beaten publicly and in some instances executed by hanging. Thomas Macy understood that the escalating Puritan bigotry threatened the freedom of all colonists. He observed this firsthand when a law was passed making it a misdemeanor for anyone other than an ordained minister to preach on the Sabbath. The law was made to restrain him from preaching to the local Baptist community in the absence of a minister on Sundays. For defying the law Thomas was required to appear before the magistrate and pay a fine which led him to pull up stakes and leave the Massachusetts Bay Colony. Early in 1659 he and several like-minded men began working on a plan to purchase the island of Nantucket, then under the jurisdiction of New York as a home and safe haven from Puritan dominance. This purchase was recorded by deed in July of that year, and plans were made to emigrate the following spring in time to plant crops.

Since coming to the aid of Quakers was a crime in Massachusetts, Macy's plans were unexpectedly accelerated. As the story goes, Kate's ancestor provided temporary shelter to several traveling Quakers during a heavy rainstorm. A Puritan neighbor brought his actions to the attention of the magistrate; rather than appear before the court Macy sent a letter explaining what had occurred. He explained that he had not known with certainty that the four men were Friends and stressed that the strangers were on his premises for less than an hour and few words were exchanged. Despite this, helping any Quaker was a crime. The letter of explanation may have saved Macy from prison, but he was fined thirty shillings and ordered to be admonished by the governor. He paid his fine and suffered the governor's admonition but vowed privately that this circumstance would never be repeated.

As noted by Silvanus Macy, his ancestor left his home in Salisbury because "he could not in justice to the dictates of his own conscience longer submit, to the tyranny of the clergy and those in authority."[3] History records that two of the four "sheltered" Quakers, William Robinson, a London merchant, and Marmaduke Stephenson, a Yorkshire man, were hanged in Boston at the end of October for the crime of following the Quaker faith. Once they learned this, Macy and his fellow Baptists were shaken. The small band of Nantucket-bound travelers were moved to make their break months ahead of schedule, setting out for Nantucket Island, some twenty-five miles off Cape Cod in stormy October seas. Accompanying Thomas and Sarah Macy and their five young children were Edward Starbuck, a twelve-year-old boy named Isaac Coleman, and Tristam Coffin. Macy, Starbuck, and Tristam's father were three of the original purchasers of Nantucket. Macy family legend relates that at the height of the storm Sarah Macy became hysterical, fearing for the lives of her children. Her husband was said to have banished her below deck for the duration of the voyage with the words, "Woman, go below and seek Thy God, I fear not the witches on earth or the devils in hell."[4]

The lives of Thomas Macy and his countless descendants were changed forever with the purchase of Nantucket on "2 July 1659." Macy and eight other men acquired the island from a "cousin," Thomas Mayhew of Martha's Vineyard. It has been recorded that they paid him with thirty pounds sterling and a pair of beaver hats, one for himself and one for Mrs. Mayhew. His agreement with the "First Purchasers" retained Mayhew as a tenth proprietor. At that time Mayhew, who had acquired his holdings from an agent for Lord Sterling, lived on Martha's Vineyard and used the land on the western end of Nantucket as a grazing place for sheep. The Macys were the first white family to settle on the island, a crescent-shaped spit inhabited by some 3,000 friendly Indians. With the natives' help, the newcomers survived the winter, living in crudely fashioned dwellings. When their provisions ran out they subsisted on plentiful fish and waterfowl and watched for signs of spring when they expected to welcome ten additional purchasers and their families at Madaket Harbor.

By the second generation, the Macy family was firmly established at Nantucket. It was in the third generation that carpenter John Macy and his wife Judith Worth joined the Religious Society of Friends along with many other early Nantucket settlers. Earlier, the Macy family tree had divided, creating healthy new branches including the one which eventually bore the well-known dry goods merchant Roland H. Macy. Roland and Kate were distant cousins; she had no direct relationship to Macy's Department Store, as would one day be incorrectly reported.

Kate's great-great-grandfather (generation five) was Jonathan Macy, husband of Rose Pinkham Macy and the first mariner in the family. He commanded a coasting vessel that transported whale oil produced on the island as well as sperm oil candles. These products fouled the air so completely that only the strongest sea breeze could provide relief from the stench. Despite the rank nature of the product, the sperm whale was pursued for two main reasons. First, the oil burned brightly, and second, it was an excellent lubricant. Furthermore, the spermataceti, found in the mammal's head (originally mistaken for the whale's sperm, hence the name), produced high quality candles. They were exported to England, creating a successful American industry. The sperm whale held another valuable prize within its bowels—ambergris—desired for a perfume fixative and considered as rare as gold. Whalers had access to two additional by-products of the mammoth beasts they pursued: whalebone and baleen. The baleen became a particularly profitable commodity due to its pliable and comb-like nature, and it was used for corset stays. To the detriment of their physical health women including Kate and her female friends and relatives relied upon tightly laced corsets to make their waists appear wasp-thin in keeping with the fashion of the time.

Jonathan Macy was a substantial ship owner and merchant, and he was further enriched through his extensive real estate holdings. His success made it possible for him to purchase a variety of items in high demand on the home island as well as gifts for his loyal and hard-working wife. During Kate's childhood her grandmother Eliza Macy served tea from a sterling silver pot that was handed down from her mother-in-law Rose, who received it from her husband on their twenty-fifth wedding anniversary. It was engraved "to Rose Pinkham from her husband Jonathan Macy" and dated 1803.[5]

As a fairly young man, Kate's great-grandfather Josiah was known to be a preeminent sea captain with a lucrative worldwide cargo trade. Like many Quaker merchants of his era, he had launched his business with his father's financial backing. Having "cut his teeth" in the Philadelphia and Baltimore trade, at the age of twenty-one (already a husband and father) Josiah loaded his first vessel, as a one-quarter partner, and set sail for Marseille. He learned how to do business in foreign ports and how to make a profitable sail. His success meant that he could be off on long and unpredictable journeys, leaving his growing family behind, as was common on the island.

His wife, Lydia Hussey Macy, and the other women of Nantucket generally took a great deal of responsibility for managing their homes, families, and island affairs. Between 1805, the year when she married and became the mother of Kate's grandfather and 1825, Lydia Macy bore nine children, two of which died as babies. She reared them on her own as her husband plied the oceans and visited such exotic ports as Calcutta, Madras, Cadiz and Madeira, building faster ships all the while. The decade between 1820 and 1830 represented the most flourishing condition of shipping in the history of the United States, and Captain Macy put his heart and soul into it, building the *Orbit*, the *Isaac Hicks*, the *Silvanus Jenkins*, and the *Diamond*. When he took charge of the *Isaac Hicks* sailing to Liverpool via Charleston, his younger brother Henry assumed command of the *Diamond* filled with cargo, pleasure passengers, and crew and bound directly for

Liverpool. Theirs was a thriving international business. Nevertheless, it was a business with potentially tragic consequences as when an unfortunate wife or mother received the news of a shipwreck involving her loved one. Kate's ancestors were not immune.

Captain Josiah Macy had purchased the *Diamond* in 1823, "on the stocks," in partnership with his friend and business associate Samuel Hicks. Josiah first sailed her to Liverpool "in 8th month, 1823," and he continued in command of her in the Liverpool trade for one year. At 120 feet, the *Diamond* had three masts, weighed just over 500 tons, and was known for its dependable speed. It made the Atlantic crossing in a mere twenty-one days.[6] Just one year later, Macy and Hicks jointly commissioned another ship, the *Isaac Hicks*, which launched for Charleston that November with Josiah Macy in command. He was to load from there with a cargo of cotton bound for Liverpool, where he anticipated crossing paths with his younger brother Henry, to whom he had passed on the command of the *Diamond*.

The *Diamond* departed New York on December 12, 1824, with thirty-three-year-old Henry Macy at the helm, in command of his first ship. Accompanying him were thirty to forty souls, consisting of his crew and a number of wealthy passengers as well as a full cargo of cotton, potash, apples, and international mail. He left behind his young and newly pregnant wife, Caroline. Their story turned tragic on January 2, 1825, when Henry's ship ran aground off the coast of Wales. Only a mile or so from shore, the *Diamond* hit an undersea reef, the Sarn Padrig (Saint Patrick) causeway. Rescuers from a lifeboat station at nearby Barmouth saved nine people; the young captain was lost. Sadly, this was not the end of misfortune for Henry Macy's family. His wife, Caroline, died soon after giving birth to their son. The story of the *Diamond* remains alive in the minds of those who visit a certain stretch of Cardigan Bay. It has been said that hundreds of barrels of apples, an out of season delicacy being transported in the doomed vessel's cargo hold, washed ashore there. The apples were retrieved, seeds were planted, and in time an orchard sprang up. The fruit became known as the Diamond Apple, a direct cousin of the apples being transported to Liverpool on Henry Macy's ill-fated final voyage.

The loss of Henry Macy and his ship deeply affected the Macy family. Captain Josiah called the shipwreck a "very sad and melancholy loss" and lamented that a "considerable" amount of property had also been lost since the freight was not insured.[7] His mother, Rose, was devastated to lose another son to the vagaries of the sea. She still ached over the earlier loss of her twenty-three-year-old son Gorham who went down at Lima, Peru.

Surprising many of his fellow Nantucket seamen, in 1827 Josiah embarked upon what would be his final voyage. While this crossing was a commercial success, it was filled with peril, and he described it as "one of the most boisterous ones" he had ever made. He felt that the right time had come to quit the sea and told his family that "scarcely anything would induce me to undertake a new voyage."[8] And so Josiah and Lydia, their younger boys, Charles, Josiah, Francis, and John, and his mother, Rose, left Nantucket for good. On the first of the new year 1828, Josiah and his oldest son, Kate's grandfather William, commenced their New York-based shipping and commission business on Front Street. The men dedicated themselves to a steady mercantile life in New York and hoped that their new business would provide a safe and dependable future for the family.

And so having first set out for sea at age fifteen, Kate's great-grandfather switched course at the age of forty. He and his wife left Nantucket in time to witness the union of their son William and Eliza Leggett Jenkins, the daughter of the Captain's best friend Silvanus Folger Jenkins.

By the late 1820s New York City's prospects were exceedingly good. *The Evening Post* founded in 1801 by Alexander Hamilton declared,

> There is not a city in the world which, in all respects, has advanced with greater rapidity than the city of New York... Whichever way we turn, new buildings present themselves to our notice. In the upper wards particularly, entire streets of elegant brick buildings have been formed on sites which only a few years ago were either covered with marshes or occupied by a few straggling frame huts of little or no value.[9]

Twenty ships sailed regularly to Liverpool; New York City could boast unrivalled coastal trade. For a man of Captain Macy's energy and drive the possibilities must have been invigorating. In a relatively short period, New York had become the leading port of the nation with customhouse duties eclipsing those of the rival ports of Philadelphia, Boston, Baltimore, and Norfolk combined. The opening of the Erie Canal further enhanced the stature of the city as a port and transportation hub. New York, the new island home of the Nantucket Macys, was on its way to becoming both the gateway to the American West and a critical link to Europe. Josiah Macy's timing could not have been better. His original business "Josiah Macy and Son" was primarily known as a shipping and commission firm and also included a successful candle manufacturing business which thrived for decades.

The Macy's transition to New York was eased by a combination of their significant wealth and the opportunity to renew old Quaker friendships. One of Captain Macy's oldest friends Silvanus Folger Jenkins (Eliza Macy's father) had quit Nantucket late in the eighteenth century but he maintained a house there and visited his home island during the summer months where his youthful relationships continued.

Chapter 4

ONCE HIS GRANDFATHER HAD RETIRED FROM BUSINESS and the firm was passed on to his father and uncles, Josiah Jr. began his ascent at Josiah Macy and Sons.

These were the halcyon days for young Kate. Her grandparents' home on Twenty-First Street was the hub of family activity where they welcomed their sons, daughters, more than a dozen grandchildren, and numerous nieces and nephews. Her mother and aunts congregated for tea and talk almost daily, and the entire extended family dined there on Friday and again on First Day after meeting. Only Kate's Uncle Silvanus and his family did not join in; they had moved to Sodus Point near Rochester, where he had established a coal business.

Kate remembered her grandmother Eliza as a strong woman, receiving visitors graciously as she sat rod straight in a carved rosewood chair appearing immune to the weight of her cumbersome attire. The quintessential New York Quaker lady, she wore long gowns with leg-of-mutton sleeves, tulle bonnet tied beneath the chin, matching cuffs, lacy shawl, lorgnette, and a smattering of tasteful jewels, and a softly curled, powdery wig. She was not one to dine at Delmonico's or the Astor House like her husband and sons, however when she went out or celebrated a special anniversary or birthday at home, she was known to fasten on her special bonnet of pale green silk, a gift purchased by her daughter Mary in Paris.

The adults in the family taught Kate the importance of staying closely connected no matter what. If you were unable to gather in the same place, you wrote letters. Mail was delivered twice each day, and letters were the principal means of communicating news among family and friends. Even relatives who lived but a few miles apart would exchange news and information by post.

The topic of health was always center stage in her grandfather's letters. Since the Macys were long involved with commerce, banking, real estate, hospitals, and other charities, updates about these activities were commonplace as well as extensive descriptions of activities pertaining to the Friends Meetings. On the occasion of a Friends Yearly Meeting that was being held in the city, her grandfather wrote his daughter Mary that so many Friends traveled to New York and housing with host families was stretched so thin that they set up cots and easy chairs for folks right at the Meeting House. Guests were treated to hot meals, boxes full of oranges, and heaping piles of fresh strawberries, which were greatly appreciated delicacies. Visiting Friends remarked that they found their temporary accommodations better than home.

In return, constant travelers like Aunt Mary and her husband regularly sent letters to loved ones with rich descriptions of their journeys—entire mornings or evenings abroad might be dedicated to correspondence. Kate's father responded with recent news in his perfect hand. Sometimes he was somber, as when relating his cousin Anna's childbirth ordeal: "They gave her chloroform and after two hours of operation took the baby from her and it is still living, the littlest thing you ever saw, it is done up in cotton, they think they will be able to raise it up…" On other occasions his sense of humor was on display as when he mentioned Dr. Fowler's upcoming nuptials, his third trip to the altar. Josiah quipped, "I cannot see what the ladies see in him, to appreciate so much, for certainly he is not so very prepossessing in his appearance."

In his final years, her grandfather's diminishing eyesight and strength impaired his handwriting greatly. Nonetheless, he wrote cogent and thoughtful letters to his family right up until his final days. After he was gone his wife gravely missed their sweet routine of reading the daily mail. She also missed his efficient household management. Bequests in William Macy's will were so generous that household staff chose to retire rather than continue to serve his widow. Stoic as ever, she claimed that she could manage on her own. With her poor vision and years of reliance on the help of others, she was hardly capable of independence. Her daughters Mary and Cornelia insisted on securing household help so that their mother could remain in her beloved home.

As luck had it, the daughter of cousins, both of whom practiced medicine, was available to serve as Eliza's companion. The young woman, Eleanor Leggett, was invited over for "a look," and it was immediately determined that she would be just fine. She lived with Kate's grandmother for almost fifteen years, until the elderly woman passed away at age ninety-three. Eleanor and her mother, Ellen Curry Leggett, a women's doctor, were outstanding examples of female competency and compassion to Kate; Dr. Ellen Leggett had studied at the Women's Medical College of the New York Infirmary while raising her family, graduating in 1873. Her daughter enjoyed a long life and a comfortable retirement, thanks to being remembered in Mary Kingsland's will in appreciation for her devoted care of Eliza. "Cousin El" died peacefully in her home, a two-room suite at the stately Hotel Shelton on Lexington Avenue, at the age of ninety. She left an account of her time with Kate's Grandmother Macy.

Eliza Macy was my grandfather Thomas Haight Leggett's niece and I spent much time with her in her home when I was a girl in my teens, after the death of her husband. When her husband died she refused to leave their home. He left generous bequests to his servants and they decided to retire on the money so Eliza engaged a good maid and two sisters to act as cook and waitress. Mary Kingsland tried to induce her mother to have a housekeeper.

I had had a bad turn of pneumonia the spring of '81 and mother, while visiting Cornelia Macy Walker that summer, told her that I had a good soprano voice and was studying singing.

Cousin Eliza, though a very strict Friend, she loved my mother and admired her, so Cornelia went to her mother and told her of me and said, "Why don't you invite Ellen's daughter to come and stay with you for the winter, thee knows thee won't go downstairs since father died, and she could have her meals in the dining room, look after the servants, see thy callers if thee didn't want to see them all and so forth."

Well Cousin Eliza said, "Tell Ellen to bring her daughter in to see me and if I like her, I'll ask her." I didn't know why I was asked to call there rather than my pretty and attractive sister Catherine, but I went, and was oh so charmed by the dainty little old lady in her beautiful heavy black silk with leg-o-mutton sleeves, tulle cap, cuffs & collar & white lace shawl. Delighted with her shrewd comments and wit I accepted her invitation with great pleasure.

While residing with Cousin Eliza I used to go over to Mother's office for advice, "How do you make fish cakes?" I went home on Saturday mornings for the weekend as that was the day her children gathered at Cousin Eliza's. She was, as she said half blind and nearly deaf, but what she didn't see and hear! After her callers had left, she had nineteen or twenty a day, I would sit with her in the evening and laugh over her comments. One of her sayings was, "When I get what I like I make a meal of it; when I don't, I make less suffice." Mary Kingsland was very good to me. I went to my first large dinner party at her home, and after to a seat in a box at the opera.[1]

Chapter 5

KATE'S FAMILY EXEMPLIFIED QUAKER SENSIBILITIES regarding charitable behavior and tender relationships. Within the Quaker home egalitarian marriage, which emphasized the important role of women, was expected, and the guiding principle within the family was love.

Kate was always depicted as a fragile child, perhaps due to her delicate build and shy demeanor. Her "Papa" was the parent who best understood her sensitive nature; her sister gravitated toward their mother.

As early as age two, Kate was afraid of people and reluctant to be far from her parents or sister. For several years her mother was obliged to give up everything and take care of Kate herself, something unheard of in her circle of privileged young matrons, and she was much criticized for giving in to Kate.

When she was about four years old, her uncle Thomas Everit persuaded her mother to join her father on a business trip and leave Kate with his family in Brooklyn. Kate would not eat or sleep. A physician was called in. He diagnosed homesickness so severe that he told the Everits that their niece might die.

Thomas Everit was understandably distressed, and like most people of his day, put his faith in medical men even when their training and expertise were fairly limited. He sent word for Carrie to come home immediately. Soon thereafter she secured a young girl to play with Kate and keep her company day in and out.

For a time, Kate wanted nothing to do with this newcomer and clung to her mother's dress in tears, hoping to regain her complete attention. Her father, the soft one, advised her mother to give in to her but Carrie held firm and began spending more time making calls and participating in charity work, often related to the Society of Friends. In her absence, Kate turned to her sister Mary, who was called Mae.

Kate continued to have difficulty separating from her parents, and over the next year or so, as the tale of Kate's aborted visit with the Everits was retold within the family, her willfulness may have been emboldened. Perhaps it was due to Kate's reluctance to be away from her mother and father that Carrie did not accompany her husband on another business trip until Kate was almost age thirteen. This was a welcome occasion for Josiah who wrote to his sister Mary Kingsland, "It was a great event for Carrie to leave the children. We have been away for a week, got back last Thursday night, had a very nice time and found them all well on our return."[1]

Quakers held a sentimental view of childhood and over time promoted the ideals of domesticity and child-centeredness that would become the norm in American society.[2] Kate and her siblings benefitted a great deal from being raised in such an environment. The Macys took to heart the principle of the loving family and positive focus on children as emphasized in the writings of the influential Quaker leader and colonial Pennsylvania proprietor William Penn. Instructing his own children about the raising of his grandchildren Penn wrote, "…free them up in a love of one and other, tell them it is the way to have the love and blessing of God upon them." He believed that parents should show children both physical and emotional love and counseled them to be "tender and affectionate…"[3] The spiritual egalitarianism that was fundamental to the Quaker faith made women important partners in child-rearing. Mothers and fathers were expected to oversee their children, and to do so with love and justice through the practice of "holy conversation." This enlightened concept was centered on the belief that children were best taught through instruction by loving parents rather than through coercion or stern discipline, the more predominant practice among other religious cultures. Quaker parents set the spiritual tone in the household through their personal example of piety and decorum. They were expected to model the values of patience, humility, simplicity, sobriety, and self-denial within the home, which was considered a haven as well as the spiritual center of family life. Mothers and fathers viewed their children as "tender plants growing up in the truth," and endeavored to love each child in equal measure.[4]

In the happy world of Kate's childhood, family members treated each other with affection and respect, and children were considered a source of delight. They were well-cared for and doted upon. The close and demonstrative nature of the Macy family is particularly evident in the affectionate terms expressed in family reminiscences and letters. In 1867, Kate's great-grandfather Captain Josiah Macy penned a lengthy missive to his grandson Silvanus who was preparing his comprehensive family genealogy. Eighty-two-year-old Josiah signed his letter, "With ardent desires for thy present and future happiness, I remain thy affectionate grandfather, Josiah Macy."[5] Letters written by family members always closed with words that were warm and loving.

The children's quips and antics became some of the most interesting features of family correspondence and conversation. The story of Kate's four-year-old "sweetheart," a little curly-haired boy who attempted to kiss her cheek at luncheon in front of the entire family became a tale repeated for years. While on a family holiday at the Profile House in New Hampshire, William Kingsland wrote to his in-laws,

> The children enjoy themselves and have first rate appetites-
> Mae can store away a good high pile of griddle cakes and Kate, for
> a little body, would make a Westchester farmer who keeps board-
> ers turn pale over the butter jar.[6]

Kate's happy family circle continued to grow. Her Uncle Will was the last to wed; he married Angelina Strange in 1866. The year before the wedding, Grandfather Macy displayed a sense of excitement as Will had gone courting at Ingleside, a Gothic Revival mansion overlooking the Hudson at Dobbs Ferry. Grandfather knew that there were "one or two young ladies to visit" and he called his only unmarried son "a regular old batch" and said he wished he would "hurry up and choose a wife."[7]

The family who owned Ingleside had little in common with the Macys; however, one of the "young ladies" twenty-year-old Angelina Sophie Strange appealed to William. Her family's story was a living example of "rags to riches." Her father Edwin and his brother Albert were the bastard sons of Mary Bruton, a cloth picker from a family of impoverished weavers in rural England. As young men the brothers moved to London, and met with some degree of financial success which allowed them to immigrate to New York. By the mid-1830s the Stranges were selling feathers, ribbons, artificial flowers and other trimmings to adorn women's hats; they had a captive market among middle and lower class women. As every Victorian woman knew hats were essential items of apparel and a worn-out hat could be inexpensively refreshed with a few simple embellishments. By providing reasonably priced trim to the masses, the entrepreneurial brothers gained a foothold in business, and in time they expanded into manufacturing fanciful silk ribbons in a Brooklyn factory before moving their business to Patterson, New Jersey, which became known as the "Silk City."

Angie Strange and her family were not Quakers, and her family lacked the pedigree and the high reputation of the Macys' typical business associates. Nevertheless, as the daughter of a wealthy merchant with a fine home the young woman was considered a suitable match for thirty-year-old William Macy, Jr. Her future father-in-law was accepting of the match and looked forward to his son's marriage. But right before the happy day, Grandfather Macy slipped and fell. While hurrying up from the cellar with an armful of Thanksgiving wine he lost his balance and went crashing down the rickety stairs. Although outwardly sympathetic, his wife was said to have quietly remarked that it was the Lord's punishment. She always maintained that the imbibing of spirits was ill-advised barring medicinal purposes. The fall caused Kate's grandfather to rip the cords around his knee and as a result he did not make it to his son William's wedding. For one known to spend much time bestowing every kindness upon the sick and injured, he proved to be an irascible patient and suffered the physical consequences of his accident for months. He never quite came to terms with missing an event that he had so long and eagerly anticipated. However, within a few years he was elated when Will and Angie started a family. Firstborn was Josephine Sophie, and then came Edwin Strange Macy. The little boy was weak from birth. It was sadly predicted that his parents could probably not raise him up to adulthood. Even though doctors and nurses were brought up to Westchester to care for him, Kate's sickly cousin died before his second birthday.

Chapter 6

DESPITE BEING RAISED IN A SECURE AND HAPPY HOME, a child of the late nineteenth century was well aware of the twin curses of illness and death. Kate saw her cousin die and also knew of the prolonged illness and death of her mother's younger sister Catherine Hicks Everit—also known as "Kate" she died when her niece and namesake was two years old. Her final days were recounted in minute detail for years to come. Catherine's infirmities and death at a young age were actually an inspiration to Kate's father who proclaimed that he would live his life differently from that time forward. He wrote about his epiphany in detail and sent his sister Mary and her husband a full account of Kate Everit's final days.

> Her last sickness was short, but eleven days. The last few days of her life, I was with her a great part of the time, they made an impression upon me I hope I may never forget to see such fortitude and happiness in one so young at such a trying hour, when all ones acts for a life are about to be tried by the mighty Judge of the living and the dead. I trust that it has been a lesson to me and that in the future I may lead a different life than I have done in the past. She has been with me in Spirit constantly since her death. She died so quietly that one could hardly tell when she stopped breathing. Since her death I have felt that I have had a great deal to be thankful for especially the preservation of my dear wife and child...I feel that it was only the hand of the divine that saved them. I pray that we may all turn our thoughts to Him and less to the world.[1]

In this letter he alludes to an experience a few months before Catherine died that also affected him greatly: a terrible scare while the family was on a summer holiday in the mountains. They were enjoying a cooling afternoon sail when circumstances caused Carrie and one of the children to fall overboard. Josiah thanked God for the preservation of his wife and daughter from a watery grave. The incident was mentioned through the years but the child was never identified by name.

The effect of these worrisome inklings of death was compounded when a particularly tragic blow struck the entire Macy family when Kate was five years old. Her Aunt Mary's son, Cornelius or "Neelie," the oldest child in Kate's generation and the apple of everyone's eye, suddenly took sick and died.

Young Kate overheard hushed conversations about the agonizing hours of the bedside vigil, Cornelius's brave final words and the state of his devastated parents and fiancée Ettie Cannon. There was a church funeral and more hushed conversation yet no one explained what had happened to the youngsters. Perhaps the adults assumed that small children would not understand or notice, but a bleak spirit had invaded the Macys' lives. Amidst the weeping and inconsolable grief, Mary Kingsland read and answered scores of condolence notes and copied prayers and psalms in a slim black journal; the crepe-trimmed black gowns with mourning jewelry so different from her usual attire were frightening to a sensitive child like Kate.

It is easy to imagine that Kate was confused and fearful. Young people, mothers in childbirth, babies in infancy, all could die; it was an occurrence too common to ignore. Death could also bring terrifying changes to a child's life. When Kate was age six the death of her Uncle Silvanus's wife Carrie Ridgway left her first cousins motherless, later to be raised by a strange new woman. Family members agreed that Sil's second wife, Juliet, could not hold a candle to his first, and his children never accepted their mama's replacement. Kate may have harbored an anxiety that she, too, could lose her mama, and that she might be replaced by a woman who allowed them to keep her daguerreotype on the bedroom dresser but preferred that they never spoke her name or asked to visit her family.

The passing of a loved one is heartbreaking for loving survivors, especially when parents lose children. Kate observed this firsthand when her Uncle Sil lost his firstborn son. In circumstances eerily similar to the death of Cornelius eight years before, Charles, age twenty, took sick and perished. His passing left Kate's family questioning anew how such things could happen.

Kate felt most secure in the cocoon of home. In her memoir she commented that she felt uneasy when a new school year resumed—

she resisted leaving home each morning. She would say goodbye to her mother over and over until her father took her by the hand and walked her the short distance to Thirty-Second and Madison Avenue to "Mrs. Roberts and Miss Walker's English and French Day School for Young Ladies and Little Girls." The academy flourished for more than fifty years, educating girls from prominent families and providing opportunities for female education unavailable to Kate's mother's generation.

On her morning treks to school, Kate and her father were accompanied by her Uncle Will Macy. Upon reaching Miss Walker's door Kate's tears would begin to flow. Despite this Kate's parents were resolute; they did not support educating their daughters at home even though many wealthy families still did so. It was fortunate, Kate admitted later, that her parents valued a modern education. She was exposed to a variety of subjects from poetry to botany to geography and realized that school helped her overcome her shyness. Nevertheless, the coming of fall was always painful for Kate as it marked the end of carefree family time in the country. The Macys always fled the oppressive heat of town from June through August visiting at the family farm in Harrison or at the popular haunts of the well-heeled including the Profile House at Franconia Notch, New Hampshire, resorts at Long Branch, New Jersey, Richfield Springs, New York, and Bar Harbor, Maine, and the Adirondack Mountains.

Into Kate's world, already well-populated by her sister Mae and many cousins, a new happiness came along when her brother was born in the early spring of 1871. He was named Valentine Everit Macy, after her maternal grandfather. Kate was eight years old and very relieved that her mama was in good health following the birth, her period of confinement having caused Kate great worry. Since Kate happened to be sick with the measles, she could not see her brother or mother for several days, but from the moment she did, he was her joy.

By the time Everit (as he was called) was born, her father was front-and-center as a petroleum refiner with an office downtown. He had been involved since he was a young man in decisions that were key to the prosperity of Josiah Macy and Sons. The industry had changed from the early days when refiners attempted to produce coal oil from an asphalt-shale process that proved too costly to be practical.

By 1859 Daniel Drake had drilled his first oil well in Pennsylvania, and as they maintained their whale oil refineries in New England, the Macy men had carefully followed the shifting trends in the oil trade. They had persisted through the Civil War and in 1867 were able to take over the bankrupt Long Island Coal Oil Company at Hunter's Point where they converted the operation to the production of kerosene from petroleum. With the reorganization, the business was renamed the Long Island Oil Company. The swampland around the property was transformed into a viable industrial sector when the area was filled in with cellar earth and street dirt from New York City, and transportation was introduced via the Long Island Railroad which had established a depot as well as regular ferry service. The new oil works' capacity increased from a daily output of 1,200 barrels to a capacity of more than 25,000 barrels a day by the late 1860s.

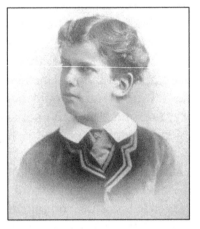

Valentine Everit Macy, age 10 *(Courtesy of the Macy Family)*

In 1868, the Macy refinery was the second largest in the country. Kate's father, a mere thirty years old, was the point person for kerosene oil production for the new family enterprise. Few men knew much about refining oil when he became involved. Josiah was named president of the Long Island Oil Company, which was a subsidiary of Josiah Macy and Sons. He was convinced that the production of clean, affordable kerosene for illuminating homes, hospitals, and businesses could change the future. Kate's father knew there was money to be made, although money was not his primary motivation. He was excited to be in on the ground floor of new technology, and no doubt, wished to prove himself in business like the Macys before him.

During those early days as the head of a young family and an up-and-coming business leader, Josiah decided the family should move to a more fashionable district of the city. Respectable families were trickling out of their neighborhood, and Carrie was not happy to be raising her family on West Twenty-Eighth Street where family homes were dwindling and being replaced by brothels. There were at least twenty-five houses of ill repute within two or three blocks of the Macy home, as confirmed in *The Gentleman's Directory of 1870,* a little black book (author unknown) that guided gentlemen to "entertainment" in the city. The directory noted the high cluster of "Dens of Iniquity" located within close proximity to the Macy home, including one situated a mere block away. The house was "presided over by Jenny Mitchell, a very agreeable and entertaining lady, who has four highly accomplished young lady boarders. With elaborate furnishings it's a first-class house."[2]

Gentleman who made use of the "Directory" could also take advantage of the guide's helpful information about condoms and cures for sexual problems, and readers were urged to be wary of the "Nymphes de Pave," comely, well-dressed "Cruisers," intent upon "robbing unsuspecting men of their all."[3]

While Kate was too young to understand, others knew that the neighborhood had become infested with immoral women who would cause decent men to sin. The tradition of taking responsibility for others (even sinners) ran deep among Quakers, and the rehabilitation of city prostitutes was aided by reputable men like the Macys who contributed to the establishment of the "House for Fallen Women" on West Houston Street. The inmates were said to possess many sins, chief of which were prostitution and the use of whiskey and opium. They were universally poor, and local business leaders believed that the women could be uplifted, saved, and set on a righteous moral path if provided with decent food and lodging, moral counseling, and religious instruction. Some female Friends may have scoffed over their husbands' support, but overall the Society of Friends viewed the fallen women as victims of poverty who presented both a moral challenge and a threat to society.

Chapter 7

JOSIAH MACY JR. CONTINUED TO FIND SUCCESS AS AN OILMAN. In an era when refined oil could be more hazardous to handle than gun powder, the Macys enjoyed a reputation for producing a safe and dependable product. Nevertheless, these were challenging times for the young petroleum industry. Rampant in-fighting existed among producers, refiners, and the railroad interests, and small operations routinely fell victim to the chaos.

By 1870, John D. Rockefeller, a man who would become closely involved with Kate's family, had entered the spotlight as an oilman. He lived in Cleveland, Ohio, a promising center for oil refining with its close proximity to Lake Erie and rail transportation. Rockefeller and his associates were in the business of buying up refineries in Ohio, Pennsylvania, and New York. To some producers he was a savior, but to many he was the devil incarnate, devouring their businesses to create one huge conglomerate. In January 1870, he and fellow corporators Henry M. Flagler, Samuel Andrews, Stephen V. Harkness, and his brother William Avery Rockefeller founded the Standard Oil Company. John D. Rockefeller was the majority stockholder. His brother William was the salesman and came east to establish a New York branch office; this is where he and Kate's father first became acquainted.[1]

Due to the size and success of the Macy petroleum operation, Rockefeller asked Josiah Macy Jr. to exchange the three refineries the Macys operated near New York City for Standard Oil stock and cash. Macy conferred with his father and brothers, and they agreed that the Rockefellers had made them a once-in-a-lifetime offer considering the lightning speed with which they were knocking down the competition. The Macy industrial and commercial enterprises held a total of five refineries in 1871, three in New York and two more in New Bedford, Massachusetts. The Macys sold only three of their five refineries to Standard to protect their finances in the event the Rockefeller business failed. In contrast to John D. Rockefeller, who was said to revel in the daily balance sheets that proclaimed his wealth, Josiah Macy Jr. and his family were modest about their holdings. Years later, it was reported that Josiah valued the three refineries that he sold to Standard Oil at $150,000. By his son Everit's estimate, that investment grew to exceed $200 million dollars over the course of the next six decades.[2]

The Rockefeller brothers admired Josiah Macy's talent and temperament. In addition to buying him out for stock and cash, they invited him to become one of their "operators." He oversaw the operation of the Devoe Manufacturing Company, serving as vice president, treasurer, and president of a company that manufactured the tin barrels critical for the safe and inexpensive worldwide transport of a product called Devoe's Brilliant Oil. The brand was far better known outside the United States since the Devoe Manufacturing Company directed its attention to the export trade—their advertising brochure was printed in twenty-one languages. The streets were lit with its clear, white steady light as far away as Jerusalem, and in Syria infant cradles were made from abandoned "Devoe's Brilliant Oil" stenciled shipping crates.[3]

Kate's father's business success made it possible for him to move his family uptown to the newly fashionable section of the city located near Fifth Avenue and the Fifties. Carrie and Josiah had been married more than fifteen years when they purchased a handsome townhouse at 18 West Fifty-Third Street; Carrie threw herself into furnishing and decorating her first marital home. In early 1876, the Macys, who delighted in such new acquisitions as a blue floral rug and a large dining table and chairs, proudly entertained the Rockefeller brothers and their wives at a special housewarming dinner. Nevertheless, Josiah did not feel fully confident about his earnings, and since he was never one to show off he did not maintain a staff. On the day of the dinner party he "borrowed" his sister Mary's servants and took it upon himself to shovel the snow off his roof. The Rockefeller brothers held Kate's father in high esteem; they admired his intelligence and strong morals. Some fifty years after Josiah Macy's death, Kate's brother Everit was sipping tea with John D. Rockefeller at his home at Pocantico Hills in New York when the older man said,

"No finer man ever lived than your father." He also told Everit that he always kept a picture of Josiah Macy Jr. on his dressing table. The Macy-Rockefeller family friendship remained an important one throughout Kate's lifetime.[4]

Kate's father worked day and night to make the Devoe enterprise a success. The operation was expected to run at capacity, and this presented Josiah with a tremendous and complex challenge due to the multitude of operations occurring simultaneously along the extensive waterfront site of the oil works. The "Devoe Brilliant Oil Works" was comprised of brick buildings, smokestacks, storage sheds, and docks, and was connected to Hunter's Point by an iron drawbridge. The dock itself was large enough to accommodate the loading of several vessels at once. In addition, fleets of lighters (barges) and steamboats were typically lying in wait to haul Brilliant Oil to vessels anchored by the docks of other businesses nearby. Here the petroleum was refined and then packed into the containers produced in the company's metal can factory, which turned out thousands of tin cans each day. An advertising card of the period described Devoe as occupying about "fifty lots of ground at Hunters Point," at that time considered to be the refined petroleum capital of the United States. Josiah was understandably concerned about the issue of safety at the works due to the highly volatile nature of refined oil, and he put tremendous stock in the soundness of the tin transport barrels that were produced in the can factory. Nevertheless, in the spring of 1876, his brother-in-law William Kingsland, who was traveling in Mexico with his wife, Mary, alerted him about the possibility of problems with the Devoe cans.

Kingsland wrote,
St. Charles Hotel
New Orleans, March 24, 1876

I noticed at Vera Cruz piled up in front of my hotel window about 500 cases of Devoe Manufacturing oil—landed from the steamship "City of Mexico"—many of the oil cans exposed—the boxes having been broken and cans much bent and quite a good deal of oil on the pavement from leakage.[5]

Josiah Macy was burning the candle at both ends, and this news was a cause for great concern. Furthermore, as Devoe and Standard Oil stock soared he appeared to be uneasy, and he wrestled with his recent material success. In a letter written in April 1876 he wrote,

> I think of it every day, how much I have been blessed, or rather how prosperous I have been. I hope & pray that I may not be carried away with it, and that I may make good use of it—I find it requires one to be constantly on the watch—or else your mind gets carried away with it—that business and making money becomes your first thought.[6]

Despite his discomfort Josiah remained committed to his around the clock labor. Throughout 1876 he served as president of Devoe, worked on legislation related to the oil industry in Washington, D.C., and traveled to Philadelphia where he represented the oil industry at the Philadelphia Centennial Exposition. The Exposition and her father's involvement figured prominently in Kate's memories of that time.

The Centennial Exposition of 1876 was designated as both a celebration of one hundred years of American Independence, and an international exhibition of the arts, manufacturing, and products of the soil and mines. Kate's father helped to organize the massive American and international oil competition entries which included such diverse products as toilet soaps, varnishes, salts, inks, machinery for sugar production, chemical and pharmaceutical preparations, coal tar products, commercial fertilizers, and every manner of oil-related product from Italian olive oil to American petroleum. Josiah's company which was among scores of entrants in the competition under the sub-category "Oils, Soaps, Candles and Illuminating Gases" was awarded a Centennial Commendation for its high-test oil and ingenious secure oil can lids.[7]

Josiah was among more than 200,000 people in attendance when President U.S. Grant addressed the crowd at the grand opening of the Centennial Exposition at noon on Wednesday, May 10th, 1876. The highlight of the opening ceremony was a one-hundred gun salute and the raising of the Stars and Stripes by the president. Thereafter, he set in motion the massive Corliss steam engine, the exhibition's anchor and centerpiece, in Machinery Hall. At 650 tons, it was the largest engine ever built and specifically designed to provide the power for all the machinery in the Hall. When the levers were engaged, the belts and shafts quivered before moving in all directions, which caused the crowd to go wild with shouts and applause.

Kate's father spent the next several days in Philadelphia
conferring with dignitaries and international leaders in business and
manufacturing. Although the official purpose of the Centennial
Exposition was to celebrate the one hundredth anniversary of the
signing of the Declaration of Independence, the fair was nothing less
than a nineteenth century consumer spectacle and the exhibitions
sprawled over almost 300 acres in Philadelphia's leafy Fairmount
Park. The majority of the space showcased Yankee ingenuity. In all
there were five large pavilions and 250 smaller ones. Some 30,0000
businesses exhibited their wares including the Remington Typewriter
Company, whose pioneering invention, the typewriter, was operated
by a foot treadle and available for the princely sum of $125. A
Remington "type-writer" employee stood ready to prepare a letter for
any visitor with fifty cents to spare.[8]

When Kate's father returned home from the Exposition he was in
a state of exhaustion. Nonetheless, he was enthusiastic about taking
his entire family to the fair in September.

And so an impressive party of Macys set out for the Philadelphia
Centennial Exposition on September 11, 1876. Among them were
Kate's parents and grandparents, her sister and brother, Everit's nurse,
Carrie's maid, and Josiah's siblings and their wives. The latter group
was comprised of Will and Angie and their little girl Josie, Cornelia
and Ike Walker and their son Willie, the Kingslands, and a cousin
Mary Smith, and assorted maids, eighteen in all. It had been an
oppressively hot summer, and even though it was mid- September, the
heat would not quit. Nevertheless, Kate and her sister found the train
trip thrilling, and they whipped their delicate lady's fans about with
abandon in an effort to circulate the close air within the car. Years
later Kate remarked that she was an exceedingly fortunate child in a
multitude of ways. Foremost, she acknowledged the sheltering love of
her family, and she was keenly aware of her privilege. For example,
even as a child she traveled in comfort and lodged at fine hotels. As
people of means, the Macys would enjoy a trip in a dustless reserved
car with comfortable upholstered seats and an atmosphere of peace.

The Macys' first impression of the Exposition was formed as
soon as they arrived at the newly constructed Centennial Depot
located directly across from the fair's main gate. They took in the
imposing bunting draped structure, flags flying aloft from rooftop

towers. The crowds were thick but the Macys, among a throng of 80,000 who visited during the month of September (which honored New York State) were met by livery drivers at the ready to transport the party and their considerable baggage to the exclusive Transcontinental Hotel, just a stone's throw from the Exposition's entrance.

As a young girl enthralled at the prospect of spending five days at the Centennial Exposition, Kate may not have been aware of her father's concerns about exposing his family to the crowds they encountered. His apprehension regarding the general sanitation of the city was related to a stay in Philadelphia the previous April when he had been particularly disturbed by the "table" at his hotel which he described as "awfull...dirty waiters, dirtier plates and the dirtiest eatery we found anywhere." However, he was subsequently convinced that conditions at Philadelphia had improved and that the "Quaker City" was a safe destination for those who stayed at the more fashionable hotels. His choice of the Transcontinental Hotel placed Kate's family in the lap of luxury. One of eight hotels adjacent to the park, the triangular building was constructed and elegantly furnished specifically for the Exposition at a cost of more than $250,000; the daily room rate of five dollars was far out of reach for the average fairgoer. This exclusivity reassured Josiah that his family would be protected from tainted water and food and insalubrious guests. Despite Josiah's desire to keep his family healthy and shield them from the tumble of the crowds, it would have been difficult for Kate and the other youngsters to resist the wide variety of treats offered at the fair. Sugary popcorn balls, Hires Root Beer (which Charles E. Hires, a Philadelphia Quaker introduced to the public by dispensing free samples), and tin foil wrapped bananas (an uncommon fruit in North America in 1876) were among the more popular novelties.

It should have been reassuring to the family that on the front page of the daily *Centennial Journal* Dr. William Pepper, director of the Medical Bureau of the Exposition, stated that the city had none of the special conditions known to induce illness, such as imperfect drainage or impure drinking water. He concluded that Philadelphia was the healthiest city in the world as it absorbed so many visitors, and yet faced few apparent health problems. As the adults read this report they might have noticed that Josiah suddenly lacked his characteristic vitality. His cheeks looked sunken, and flecks of gray dappled his luxurious muttonchops and beard.

Despite concerns over her husband's lack of vigor, Kate's mother joined the other women to tour the exhibits of porcelain and precious metals and gems. Tiffany and Company created unique silver pieces for the Exhibition including metalwork featuring American Indian motifs and a Grecian vase commissioned to honor the poet William Cullen Bryant. It was intricate, delicate and yet powerful, and claimed attention from men and women alike. In 1876 Tiffany was best known for the production of silver and gold items manufactured in Newark, New Jersey, not for the glass and jewelry that would become its hallmark. Nevertheless, many other companies displayed gems galore including diamonds that were newly available due to the expansion of mining in Africa. The centerpiece of the diamond display was a necklace and earring set of perfectly matched stones rumored to be for sale for $100,000. Carrie and her sisters-in-law also examined the popular displays of antique European lace. In the hands of a skilled seamstress these delicate wonders would transform an ordinary collar or bodice into a one-of-a-kind garment. Such laces were destined to become family heirlooms, passed down from mother to daughter to embellish wedding gowns and floor length bridal veils. Kate's mother's "laces" remained in the Macy family for generations. Her sister Mae's rose point lace wedding veil was refashioned and in use by Macy descendants until the 1960s.

Chapter 8

KATE ENJOYED HER VISIT TO THE EXPOSITION; however, her sense of excitement over the wonders she witnessed was overshadowed by illness running through the family. Almost everyone in the family returned to New York with a bowel ailment. Her father had been right to question the sanitation at the fair, and while his family recovered quickly, he did not. William Kingsland was especially worried and implored Josiah to slow down and rest.

The Macy family physician, Dr. John Gray, determined that Josiah had contracted typhoid fever in Philadelphia. He visited the house on Fifty-Third Street twice a day, but his patient's condition declined, and by the beginning of October he was dangerously ill. Dr. John Gray felt that Josiah had a mild case of the fever; nevertheless, his body was unable to fight it. He told Kate's mother that although the fever had broken, "he is worn out, as he has lived as much in his thirty-eight years as most men of eighty."[1] On October 3, the family united to hold vigil at Josiah's bedside; he died at home two days later. His funeral was held there in accordance with the simple Quaker practice without clergy or a service, or the benefit of a choir or incense. Kate's father was eulogized briefly by John D. Wright, a meeting elder. A prayer was offered, and then his body was delivered to the Grand Central Depot where a special train had been reserved to convey his coffin up to Woodlawn Cemetery for burial in the Macy family plot.

Josiah Macy's death, at age thirty-eight was a stunning blow to his close-knit family and a particular sorrow to Kate who said, "The sun will never shine again for me."[2] She was thirteen at the time but recalled that her beloved father's passing changed her almost overnight; she took on new responsibility and commented that her Papa's death made a woman of her.

After her husband's funeral Carrie penned a rare letter to her children to communicate her husband's "happy state of mind" at the time of his death. She wrote that on Sabbath morning, the first of October, four days before he died,

> He woke in a very excited manner told me to send for the Doctor as quick as possible. I tried to quiet him as I thought he had just awakened out of a sound sleep and did not know what he was about, but I soon found he knew what he wanted much better than I did. I rushed to the front room to call Mother and upstairs for the girls to send them for the Doctor and William Henry, when I went back to the room I said to him, "It is time for you to take your medicine," he replied that he did not want to take it, for it was of no use. I then said to him how do you know it is of no use? His reply was "because I have seen my Heavenly Father and he told me so." This he said in such a manner and tone of voice that I felt convinced that he knew more than those around him. "Yes, Carrie, I have seen Nealie Kingsland and he is a happy Angel in Heaven, I hope you will tell Mary so. When I was a child my Mother taught me to tell the truth and to keep a clean heart and I have always tried to do it, now God has called me and I am resigned. I am not afraid to die.[3]

According to family members, Josiah Macy's final words were, "The telegraph is broken."

The following day the newspaper reported,

> Josiah Macy Jr. President of the Devoe Manufacturing Company, No. 80 Beaver Street, died yesterday morning of typhoid fever. The deceased, who was well known in business circles, was a member of the Produce Exchange. He contracted the fever while on a visit to the Centennial, at one of the hotels where the drainage was defective.[4]

Carrie Macy suffered tremendously as a young widow. Her husband had been everything to her, as she was to him. After he died, she thought less about herself and spent more time doing for others. Family members considered her to be a capable businesswoman; she managed the mortgages on properties that her husband had amassed, figured out household expenses to the penny, and still managed to make regular contributions to the many charities she supported. She was comforted by letters of sympathy and was consoled by the Rockefeller brothers, who promised to keep a watchful eye on their former partner's young family, as well as by the sentiments expressed in the large collection of "Minutes" she had received and displayed in their dark leather folios in the parlor. Minutes were tributes to the deceased and came from organizations and businesses such the U.S. Produce Merchants Exchange, the Leather Merchants, and schools, hospitals, and banks, all places where her husband had served as an officer or board member. For the family these elaborately decorated tributes were tangible evidence of Josiah Macy's high level of achievement in both business and the community, despite his short time on earth.

Early in the new year of 1877, Kate was stunned to learn that her sister, who had turned sixteen the month after their father died, was to embark on "The Grand Tour" with the Kingslands. Kate understood that Mae was selected for special treatment because the Kingslands were her godparents and that with their mutual feelings of grief over the loss of Josiah, Aunt Mary thought that her older niece would make a suitable travel companion. Kate's sister, aunt, and uncle set sail for Liverpool on a frigid January day on the White Star steamer *Adriatic*. This was Mae's first ocean voyage; she would spend the next six months touring the great cities of Europe. Kate was envious and wondered who might come and rescue her from the unhappiness she felt without her beloved Papa.

Newsy letters from Europe exacerbated Kate's sense of being alone and adrift. She read that her sister was the beneficiary of exciting adult experiences. Mae wrote of drinking champagne in Rheims on First Day (which tactfully was not reported to Grandma Macy), and visiting the elegant gambling Casino in Monaco. On an extended stay in Paris she studied French with a tutor and was pampered by "Auguste the Court Coiffeur" who reigned at Rue de la Paix 7 next to the House of Worth. Hairdressers could be found on nearly every street in Paris, and "Auguste" was among the finest. William Kingsland wrote and told his in-laws that after Auguste elaborately styled her tresses Mae was "thrilled with the look" because she "thinks she looks eighteen."[5]

Kate keenly felt that she and her sister were drifting further and further apart, and she was dismayed that Mae was having the time of her life when the folks at home were in mourning. Uncle William affectionately referred to his wife and niece as "the girls"[6] and said, "My Mary keeps quite French in figure, Mae is getting quite Dutch."[7] Kate interpreted this to mean that her sister was emerging as a buxom and mature young woman while at age thirteen she was not at all developed and could pass for an even younger girl. For the first time in her life she experienced jealousy and was envious of the fine clothes that Aunt Mary selected for Mae—dresses, a winter cloak, gloves, shoes, and a dressing gown, which prompted William to quip that his wife and niece "pulled so hard at the purse strings."[8] However, Kate's envy was somewhat tempered when she learned that despite their gay activities her family's sadness over the loss of her father had not abated and that Mae and Mary offered each other much needed comfort and understanding. William Kingsland wrote,

> I hope that you will find Mae much improved after our journey and that the time spent with us has been of no disadvantage to her…she feels herself a young lady now… I hope she may be more than ever a great comfort and support to her mother.[9]

After months of resenting her sister, Kate understood that despite the pretty trappings and fine experiences, a dark cloud followed her loved ones—Kate's aunt and uncle were also in mourning and rushing off on the grand tour could do just so much to alleviate their pain.

While her sister toured London, Paris, Venice, Vienna, and Frankfort on Main, Kate dealt with her sadness by spending more time with her Macy grandparents. She visited them as often as possible for she could not bear to witness her mother's sadness. Kate saw that everyone dealt with their grief over Josiah's death in their own way. For example, her grandmother felt it very intensely but like a good follower of Christ she was reconciled to his loss. She preferred to mourn at home; nevertheless, she appreciated receiving guests in her parlor. Eliza's way did not work for her husband. Although he missed his son profoundly, he was up and out the door early each morning to attend to his numerous affairs, as was his custom.

Already a septuagenarian, Grandfather maintained a schedule so rigorous that it would have left a far younger man gasping for breath. He was an officer at several banks as well as for the Second Avenue Railroad Company, and he served on multiple boards such as the Society for the Prevention of Cruelty to Children and the Children's Aid Society, and he never hesitated when asked to serve as an estate executer. However, William Macy was most passionate about his work with hospitals, including the New York Society for the Ruptured and Crippled, Roosevelt Hospital, and the Society of the New York

Hospital. He had most enjoyed his years of hospital involvement when he had worked side-by-side with Kate's father, whom he was grooming to fill his shoes.

The winter of 1877 was bitterly cold in New York City, and while her grandmother remained indoors accepting callers, Kate accompanied her grandfather around town while he tended to his charity work. As president of the Society of New York Hospital, the second oldest hospital in the country having been chartered during the reign of King George III, he was occupied with the final preparations for the opening of a new hospital building. The seven-story edifice was designed by the architectural firm of George B. Post whose great-uncle was the hospital's longtime attending surgeon Dr. Wright Post. This led some to assume that nepotism was at work. Nevertheless, William Macy insisted that the infirmary be state-of-the-art in every respect and was pleased with Post's architectural plan. Innovations such as steam heat, well-lit wards, elevators, and fireproof construction transformed his design into a first-rate hospital. Privileged patients who could pay for their hospital stay had access to accommodations that emulated lodgings in fine hotels. Spacious rooms with special seating areas for visitors were decorated with attractive carpets and lamps and floor to ceiling windows; papered walls were hung with artwork and mirrors. In contrast, patients without means were housed in Spartan wards; however, they were well cared for and often treated without charge.

The new hospital was located on Fifth Avenue between Fifteenth and Sixteenth Streets. During her visits Kate would have been aware of the construction of a passageway in the rear of the building that connected the hospital to the former Thorne mansion on the Sixteenth Street side. This was where the hospital administrative offices, medical library and museum, and nurse training school were to be located. As she became better acquainted with her grandfather's work Kate considered how she might also come to the aid of the infirm. During this period opportunities for women to study medicine and nursing were on the rise. In 1877 approximately 1,000 women doctors practiced medicine in the United States, and as a result of the success of British nurse Florence Nightingale, cities throughout the country were launching professional nurse training programs.

At age fourteen Kate requested the opportunity to go to the new hospital to read and visit with patients. William Macy had taken his granddaughter to the hospital's grand-opening celebration in March of 1877 so she felt a part of all that he and her father had worked hard to achieve. Since her father had also devoted himself to hospital work and served as president of the New York Hospital for Women (which managed the first homeopathic medical college for women), Kate may have assumed that her family would support her interest in helping the sick. To her disappointment, however, her mother and grandfather denied her request, contending that she was too delicate to spend time among the sick. It is impossible to know exactly why Kate was not permitted to help at the hospital but in all likelihood, having so recently lost Josiah, William and Carrie may have feared that Kate would become ill through exposure to illness. Furthermore, they probably felt that it was inappropriate for a young girl of Kate's class to spend time among strangers in the hospital. Kate accepted their pronouncement without argument but she was devastated. Even at a tender age she recognized that by helping others to heal, she could also heal herself. This philosophy became one of her guiding principles. It is also likely that exposure to her family's charitable work with the sick inspired her future interest in health-related advocacy and philanthropy.

The year after the hospital opened, journalist W.H. Rideing lavished praise upon it and called the institution "noteworthy for its magnificence" and said that everything from floor to ceiling was "new, clean and bright" with air that was "fresh and pure," even in the notoriously noxious surgical wards. He described the building's pleasant surroundings, the sunshine streaming through "big, generous windows," and related that even when Jack Frost had paid a visit the place exuded the "balmy mellowness of a temperate summer" with plants and flowers in bloom and "fountains gurgling, spurting, and bubbling."[10] George B. Post and William Macy could congratulate themselves on the success of their creation—the hospital was called an Elysium where "the poorest patient may enjoy luxuries vouchsafed seldom to any but the rich."[11]

Once it was up and running and she was denied further involvement, Kate found herself mired in unhappiness. Life without her father was very difficult. As she struggled with her grief, Carrie's world revolved around taking care of her children, and she focused her efforts on five-year-old Everit. Once Mae returned from her Grand Tour Kate found her to be a different person, as if the trip abroad had changed her: She had developed an interest in men and preferred to spend time gossiping about romance with other young women who were more sophisticated than her sister. Kate felt left out. It came as a relief when the Kingslands proposed a family trip across the West, and Carrie agreed that a change of scenery would be beneficial to everyone.

In 1878 a western voyage was considered daring and rustic even for well-heeled and experienced travelers like the Kingslands. William Kingsland provided a bird's-eye view of the family's ambitious journey in his diary,

> March 7, 1878, Thursday. Mary, myself, Victoria, Carrie, Mae, Kate Everit & Maggie left New York via Pennsylvania and Fort Wayne Railroad to Chicago and Via Chicago and Northwest Union & Pacific Central Railroad to San Francisco—visiting the Geysers, Southern California, Yosemite, Salt Lake, Colorado & Denver, Manitou, Colorado Springs, Georgetown & via Chi Burlington to Chicago & Niagara Falls, spent 3 days at Sodus Point & arrived Incleuberg Saturday, June 15—Carrie & family went to 21St New York.

Kate's coast-to-coast trek covered thousands of miles and exposed her to the rugged beauty of the western United States. She was entranced by the splendor of the Sierra Nevada Mountains and noted that she would "never forget the superb, awe-inspiring view as one enters the Valley called rightly, 'Inspiration Point'...it was a wonderful trip, and all I saw has remained very fresh in my mind, particularly the marvelous Yosemite Valley which is beyond any description."[12]

In those years itinerant photographers traveled from place to place nationwide. They lugged their heavy equipment in the hope of immortalizing the likenesses of Americans at home or on holiday. Although she had no photograph to commemorate the majesty of the Yosemite Valley, Kate cherished a picture that captured her and her siblings resting outdoors. It is a tangible reminder of the paradox of the affluent Gilded Age easterner "roughing it" in the western

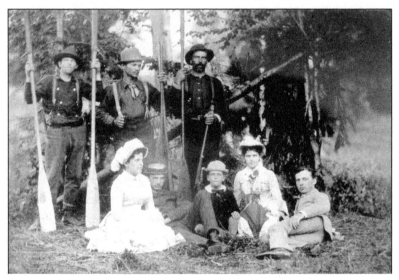

During their western tour in the spring of 1878: Pictured in the front row, from left are: Mae, Howard Willets, Everit, Kate, and an unidentified travel companion *(Courtesy of the Macy Family)*

wilderness. Three raw mountain guides stand stiffly behind a group of youthful New Yorkers. The men clutch long, wooden oars, one holds a rifle. They are lean and wear rough cut shirts and threadbare trousers. In contrast, Kate, her siblings, and two young men are seated on a carpet of grass and straw under a canopy of trees. The girls wear hats and are clad in white from head to toe as if they are going to a garden party. Mae's large bonnet is festooned with elaborate plumage; the bodice of her virginal dress is buttoned up almost to her chin. She looks away from the camera and appears to be uneasy. Kate, on the other hand, looks confident and stares intently at the camera, unaware that one of the mountain guides appears to assess her with hungry eyes. Her dress is covered with ruffles and a dainty parasol is perched on her lap. The sisters are flanked by a pair of fashionable young men and young Everit, whose attire is that of a proper city boy: straw hat, starched white shirt with ribbon tie, knickers and leather boots. The image of the mountain men and the city sophisticates is one for the ages.

Since Carrie Macy perennially suffered from digestive problems and rheumatism, William Kingsland was sure to incorporate stops at a few health resorts on the party's homeward trek. Nineteenth century travel writer Samuel Bowles popularized the notion that miraculous cures could be achieved by bathing in the hot sulfur springs at Manitou near Pike's Peak in the new thirty-eighth state of Colorado. There Kate was first exposed to a large congregation of wealthy health seekers who called themselves "invalids," a term that did not carry a stigma. Carrie and Mary Kingsland further indulged in the water cure at the New Avon Bath Spring, advertised as the "Western Saratoga," while they visited with Silvanus Macy and his family at Sodus Point, New York.[13]

Chapter 9

KATE'S LIFE TOOK A DRAMATIC TURN WHEN SHE WAS AGE SIXTEEN. She was still considered to have a delicate constitution and whether she truly was unusually delicate is questionable based on her active life and robust appearance in photographs of this time. Kate was a physically active girl and said that she loved "all kinds of sports—tennis, horse-back riding, croquet and bowling" where she chose "the largest ball in the alley."[1] She felt that nothing was too much for her to undertake and was known to play croquet in her riding habit to save time between activities. Nevertheless, the family physician advised Carrie to take her daughter out of school and have her tutored at home, and she complied. It is possible that the word delicate was used to indicate Kate's sensitive nature and to convey what we understand today to be typical changes in behavior due to hormonal production associated with puberty. We do not know whether Kate disputed her mother's decision; however, in this era doctors widely believed that too much schooling would overstrain a young woman's "delicate" constitution and possibly interfere with her future development, and Carrie would have ascribed to this ideology. Fortunately for Kate, who had reservations about being separated from her classmates, her mother engaged an excellent tutor, Miss Julia E. Nott; she proved to be an important and influential figure in Kate's life. The women maintained a warm friendship for forty-five years, and Miss Nott was also close to Carrie, who bequeathed her $75,000 when she died.

Julia Nott brought the benefits of a resilient life to her new position. She was born in Cleveland, Ohio; an only child, her father died when she was eight years old. Thereafter, she and her mother moved east and reunited with family in Rutland, Vermont where Mrs. Nott found employment as a housekeeper in the home of Martin and Frances Porter Everts. The couple was well-known in town: Martin Everts was an attorney, and local official, and his wife was from an upper-crust Rutland family. Julia and her mother resided with them in a commodious Italianate house on the corner of West and Lincoln Streets. The Everts never recovered from the loss of their three young children, and Julia, who was bright and curious, added a welcome element of cheer to their home. They took an interest in her education ,and after she graduated from Rutland High School in 1869, she enrolled at Middlebury Seminary, with her sights set on a teaching career.

Miss Nott arrived in New York, accompanied by her mother, as an unmarried woman of twenty-six years with tutoring experience and excellent references. She and Kate developed a warm bond, and ultimately Kate commented that she felt that she learned much more during the two years of study with Miss Nott than she learned all her years at school from seven to sixteen. She said her tutor taught her about "life itself which was more valuable than anything else."[2] This sounds quite exemplary; however, it is entirely possible that Julia's instruction fell somewhat short in one regard. Her tutor was aware of Kate's budding femininity—like her sister Mae she had become attracted to young men—and she was pretty, coquettish, and naïve. Since Julia Nott had limited personal experience with men, her advice on matters of the heart was limited and may have been derived from the stories about romantic entanglements in the magazines and works of fiction that she and Kate read.

The year 1881 marked what would be remembered as an irrevocable turning point in Kate's life: Within just a few months she celebrated her eighteenth birthday, adopted a new religion, and met her future spouse.

It was not unusual for young women of Kate's class to be feted at elaborate coming-out parties when they turned age eighteen. However, the Macys' custom for marking a special occasion was understated in keeping with their Quaker ways. Kate's birthday was celebrated in the company of other women with an afternoon tea. She wore a white lace dress created especially for the occasion and complemented by a double-strand pearl choker and matching ear bobs. Her dark hair was curled softly in the front and swept up in ivory combs. To commemorate the day she visited the photography studio of Mr. J. Mora at 707 Broadway and posed demurely in her party attire. Two days later, on April 8th, 1881, she carried out a plan that was several years in the making when she was baptized as a member of Dr. Hall's Fifth Avenue Presbyterian Church.

Kate's decision to leave her Quaker faith was puzzling to those who did not know her well since both the Macys and Everits had attended Quaker Meeting for generations. Kate respected her family's long-held ties to the Religious Society of Friends, but she felt adrift after the death of her father, and she found little consolation in the Quaker tradition of silent worship. As a result, she spent several years trying out other churches, hoping to discover a more secure spiritual home.

Although her grandparents were crestfallen over Kate's decision to relinquish her membership in the Religious Society of Friends, their granddaughter was not the first in the family to do so. Beginning in Kate's parents' generation, several of her aunts and uncles left the Quaker fold when they married non-Quakers: Kate was the first to choose a new faith on her own. Her parents were among the few who remained faithful Friends, although even they were not immune to the pleasures of a Christian minister's well-delivered sermon. They attended Episcopal and Presbyterian services when they were on summer holiday and far from a Quaker Meeting House. Kate felt relieved that her mother supported her decision to join Dr. Hall's fashionable church, and although she never relinquished her membership in the Society of Friends, Carrie went so far as to purchase a "family pew" there. She viewed the Presbyterians as less ostentatious than the Episcopalians and liked the fact that Dr. Hall's congregation emphasized the importance of education and charity.

Kate's union with the Fifth Avenue Church coincided with a period of unprecedented growth for prosperous New York City congregations. Many churches founded in lower Manhattan had moved north, responding to the uptown migration of their affluent members. They erected imposing buildings with jewel-toned stained-glass windows and elegant, cushioned pews, so different from the simple Quaker meetinghouse where Kate and her family had always worshipped.

Dedicated in 1875, the Fifth Avenue Presbyterian Church exemplified those long-established New York churches that had followed its migrating congregation over the decades. Built of red sandstone and topped by an impressive steeple, it was the tallest building in the city for a time. The church's minister, Reverend Dr. John Hall, who was born in Northern Ireland, was considered one of the most prominent clergymen in the United States. When he died his obituary hailed him as the most powerful and influential minster in the country, which helps to explain how an impressionable girl like Kate fell under his spell. She saw him as an ideal minister and perhaps as a father figure. On the day that she joined Dr. Hall's Church Kate records that she sang,

"When sins and fears prevailing rise,
And fainting hope almost expires, Jesus!
To Thee I lift mine eyes,
To thee I breathe my soul's desires…"

Kate, as we have learned, was accustomed to spending summers on holiday. Like most wealthy urbanites, her family chose to escape the city heat and humidity from late June until August or September, and as a result Kate visited many well-known Victorian holiday resorts including Saratoga Springs, Martha's Vineyard, and most recently Long Branch, New Jersey, where fresh ocean breezes and a touch of presidential panache made the town a popular seaside destination for members of the upper class. In 1869 President Ulysses S. Grant spent the summer by the sea at Long Branch for which it was dubbed the nation's summer capital. Thereafter, Presidents Garfield, Arthur, McKinley, Hayes, Harrison, and Wilson also spent time there. One among them, James A.

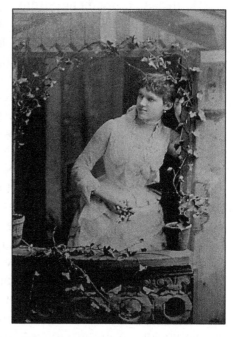

Kate, age 18 *(Courtesy of the Macy Family)*

Garfield, did not holiday at the resort town; he went there to recuperate from complications of a severe gunshot wound two months after surviving an assassination attempt on July 2, 1881. Sadly, his convalescence was short-lived; he died at Long Branch on September 18, 1881, where all of the seven presidents are remembered with a small monument overlooking the Atlantic at Seven Presidents Oceanfront Park.

While staying at Long Branch, Kate and holiday companions Lizzie and Jennie Remsen would have ambled by the sea, outfitted in navy blue frocks of loosely woven wool. Despite the heat, this was proper attire for young women at seaside resorts. The Macys lodged at the Howland House which offered luxurious accommodations and dining. Guests enjoyed everything from beignet soufflé, roasted spring chicken and ribs of prime beef to farm fresh vegetables such as new peas, stewed tomatoes, summer squash, and fried eggplant. Selections of dried fruit from California, wedges of English stilton, apple pie, and Neapolitan ice cream rounded out the menu.

A treasured memento from Kate's summer holidays was her autograph book, the *Golden Floral Album*. The number of entries from newfound friends, male and female alike is a testament to her popularity. The cover of the small book is embossed with delicate posies and flower buds and many of the pages inside have fanciful color illustrations—drawings of a cabin by a stream, flamingoes and palms, flowers, butterflies and bees. Kate's friends inscribed the pages with their autographs, good wishes, short poems, and capricious drawings such as those by friends Nannie and Carrie Paret which add a touch of whimsy to the album. Nannie's pencil drawing was called "Three little kittens, they washed their mittens" and depicts a trio of kittens dressed in trousers with large bows tied around their necks. While most of the pages are covered with innocent poems or religious messages, artwork or bold signatures, Kate received one note that stands out as being somewhat provocative for the time. An unknown acquaintance, perhaps one of her admirers, wrote, "There is nothing original in me, excepting original sin."

In June 1881, Kate and her family traveled by train and coach to the picturesque watering-hole of Richfield Springs in Otsego County, New York. The trip took almost nine hours. Carrie Macy hoped that the widely acclaimed restorative powers of the seventeen local mineral springs would relieve her chronic rheumatism. The Macys were guests at the Spring House Hotel where they joined the ranks of such socially prominent families as the Philadelphia Wanamakers, (successful dry goods merchants who may have assumed incorrectly that Kate's family was associated with the R.H. Macy store), the New York Griswolds, assorted Vanderbilts and Twomblys, and the Brooklyn Van Wycks and Polhemuses, to name but a few. The Macy entourage expanded when Carrie's mother, Beulah Everit, her younger bachelor brother Edward, a sister Anna Everit Hurlburt, and Anna's husband and brother-in-law joined them.

Carrie treated her family to holidays, and her generosity toward them was an important example to her children; however, it was beneficial to her as well. For example, with the Everits on hand at Richfield, she was assured pleasant adult companionship and in addition she expected that her brother would escort her daughters around town in place of their usual chaperone Julia Nott. Miss Nott was spending the summer with John D. Rockefeller and his family at their country place, called Forest Hill, near Cleveland. Miss Nott was serving as the children's summer tutor and governess. The comely five-foot seven-inch Julia had a decided influence on John D. Rockefeller, Jr. (a friend of Kate's brother Everit) who was smitten with her. His high regard continued through his college years as evidenced by numerous entries in his account book, which read "Flowers—Miss Nott."[3]

By the 1880s, Richfield Springs was considered a smaller and less pretentious version of Saratoga Springs. Originally known as a retreat for the lame and feeble, the legendary sulfur springs offered invalids the hope of a miracle cure. The Macy party was among a record number of health seekers in June of 1881. The local newspaper, *The Richfield Springs Mercury,* suggested that the elevated number of summer visitors was directly related to ailments associated with the previous winter's unusually severe weather. Among the Richfield guests a curious custom circulated. Some sufferers were so desperate for a cure that they carried a silver coin while taking treatments. When the coin turned black, it was said to signify that the body had become thoroughly impregnated with sulfur, a sure sign of impending relief.

Kate was happy to learn that the infirm accounted for but a fraction of the Richfield holiday population. Most cure seekers, like her mother, were accompanied by more hale and hearty family members, and Kate discovered that there was a gay side to life at

Richfield. Healthy summer guests banded together to create a small society of their own. This included a bevy of fashionable society girls and many nice-looking men from good families.

Life at Richfield agreed with Kate. She and her sister immersed themselves in the lively society of the younger set while Carrie immersed herself in a daily routine of mineral baths. The girls found that something of interest was always afoot, although occasionally something unpleasant erupted, as was the case at the end of July when a local spinster committed suicide in her home. *The Richfield Springs Mercury* described the deceased woman as "amiable" and in possession of "unusually strong intellectual powers," but stated that of late she was "greatly depressed in mind." Nevertheless, no one anticipated "the painful act by which her life was closed."[4]

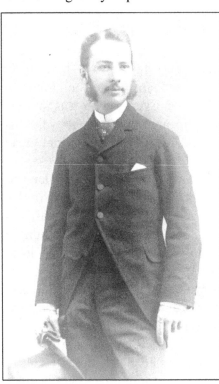

Walter Graeme Ladd, age 25
(Courtesy of the Macy Family)

In the meantime, Carrie had become so focused on her health cure that she barely noticed her daughters' comings and goings, and all the while the girls' Uncle Eddie was too intent upon his own amusement to properly assume the duties of a chaperone. As a result, Kate and Mae experienced new heights of freedom. They befriended a group of girls including Theodora Marie ("Dora") Van Wyck and Adelaide McAlpin who became Kate's lifelong friends.

The Macys had been in residence at the Springs for about one month when a handsome newcomer arrived, and both Kate and Mae took notice. The young man was from Brooklyn, and Kate's friend Dora knew him. His name was Walter Graeme Ladd, and Kate begged to be introduced. The perfect opportunity presented itself at a hotel dance called a "German," as much a parlor game as a dance and the most popular dance of the day. A master of ceremonies led dancers in a series of games set to music and awarded small trinkets to participants. The German was well-liked because young people could meet and mingle in a light-hearted atmosphere. Kate recalled that Walter Ladd was a sophisticated young man; from the moment they first linked arms on the dance floor he showed an interest in getting better acquainted. Nevertheless, there was a complication. Kate's sister Mae also sought Mr. Ladd's attention.

Walter Ladd was short and slight in stature, but he made up for these shortcomings with his handsome face and charming manners. Since he was seven years older than Kate, her sister Mae saw him as a more suitable companion for her. The girls simultaneously vied for his attention and he responded by showing an interest in both. When Mae suddenly "took ill" and retreated to her room for a few days, Mr. Ladd visited. However, most of his time was spent out and about with Kate, who was unchaperoned.

As they passed a few days together, Kate and Walter exchanged stories about their very different families. Walter told Kate that he was born in Throggs Neck, north of New York City and was raised on a dignified country estate located a stone's throw from Long Island Sound. Like Nantucket, Throggs Neck had a storied colonial history. In the seventeenth century the area was called "Throckmorton" after an Englishman with ties to Roger Williams. In 1642, Throckmorton became infamous as the site of a bloody Indian massacre where white settlers, including the minister Anne Hutchinson, were murdered.

Walter's family had settled in Throggs Neck when his father was a young man. He confided that his boyhood years at Throggs Neck were monotonous, the companionship of his three brothers being his saving grace. And he spoke kindly of his mother, Sarah, a quiet and religious woman, but said little about his merchant father. In addition, Walter explained that the Ladds had come to live at Throggs Neck through the kindness of the Ladd family "benefactor," a Scotsman named William Whitehead who owned the Throggs Neck estate and had a business office downtown. He had moved Walter's grandfather James Ladd, his wife Fanny and their children to his estate about a dozen years before Walter was born; James Ladd managed the place. Walter did not know how James and William Whitehead had become acquainted but he knew that his paternal grandfather had come from England. Despite their different backgrounds Kate was pleased to know that Walter was well-educated and had been raised in a church-going family. He told that her that he had attended Brooklyn Polytechnic Institute, was a regular church-goer, and that his younger brother was preparing for the ministry.

The Ladd family line seemed complicated to someone with a well-defined pedigree such as Kate: Walter explained that after his grandfather James died, his grandmother Fanny married family benefactor William Whitehead whom she had known for more than thirty years. When he died, Fanny inherited the bulk of her second husband's estate, more money than she had ever known. Walter further explained that he first experienced urban life at age twelve after his grandmother's death. His family joined his father's siblings in Brooklyn. Walter's aunts had wed Irish-born, Scottish-educated doctors who knew each other from their days as ship's physicians for the Cunard steamship line. Fanny's children shared her estate which included proceeds from the sale of the Throggs Neck property. This eventually made it possible for Walter's father to purchase his own home, a brownstone at 195 President Street in Cobble Hill, which is where Walter was living the summer he met Kate at Richfield Springs.

During their time together Walter told Kate about his ancestry. The account he shared was less striking than the story she could weave about the Macys and the Everits, but this did not give her pause. She was well aware that she descended from a larger-than-life clan, especially on her father's side.

Even as she began to more fully comprehend that they came from different worlds, Kate remained steadfast in her desire to pursue a romance with Walter. She knew that her mother considered a person's lineage and family connections to be of supreme importance, especially in the realm of courtship and marriage. Therefore, in anticipation of Carrie's questions and concerns, she focused on what the two families had in common. Walter revealed that he knew little about his mother Sarah Hannan Phillips Ladd's antecedents even though several distant relations lived in New York City and he was also uninformed about his paternal grandfather, James Ladd, who had died a few years before he was born. By contrast, however, he had a great deal to tell Kate about his grandmother Fanny Beach whose "Connecticut Yankee" ancestry would resonate with her mother.

Fanny Beach and James Ladd were both descended from British stock, like the Macys and Everits. However, James Ladd, the son of John and Mary Ladd and a transplant from Plymouth Dock, a naval outpost in Devonshire, England left behind few traces of his ancestry. Kate assumed that Plymouth Dock was a respectable place since "Plymouth" was part of the town's name. She pictured it populated by forthright Pilgrims, and the port of embarkation of the *Mayflower,* but this was not the case. Kate wanted to believe that Walter's paternal grandfather came from a robust maritime town, a British counterpart of the Macys' ancestral Nantucket Island. In reality, James's life in southwest England during the late eighteenth and early nineteenth century was probably quite different from what Kate imagined.

The village of Plymouth Dock, on the River Tamar, was established about 1700 as a settlement for workers employed by the Royal Navy Dockyard which had been created by the order of William of Orange a decade earlier. It was the site of the first stepped stone dry dock in Europe, and a military presence had existed there from about 1588, the time of the Spanish Armada. Over the next three centuries more than 300 naval vessels would be built at Plymouth Dock (whose name would be changed to Devonport in 1823 to distinguish it from the actual nearby town of Plymouth). By the advent of the Napoleonic War, Plymouth Dock was reportedly "honeycombed with the haunts of vice and debauchery, and had earned for itself an unenviable reputation throughout the whole kingdom for the most daring and flagrant lawlessness."[5] Of particular concern was the need to appoint a night watch since a great number of strangers and foreigners lingered about, including many Spaniards who "escorted" local women to their ships; English soldiers responded to this by attacking the Spaniards and the brawl was said to have ended with the Englishmen triumphantly retrieving the women. Plymouth Dock was also afflicted with the "sacrilegious plundering of poor-boxes" and "her lanes were infested by footpads and wandering wastrels...and outlying farmhouses were broken into at night, and produce, cattle, sheep, horses, and women were carried bodily away."[6] To make matters worse, by the end of the war with France, there was little work at the docks. It stands to reason that this state of affairs fueled James Ladd's decision to emigrate to North America. Having lived in Plymouth Dock he may well have possessed skills that would be welcomed at the bustling docks of lower Manhattan.

Like Kate's ancestors, the Beaches immigrated from "Old England" to New England during the seventeenth century. Throughout their first several generations in America the Beach men distinguished themselves as landowners, ministers and clergymen— and an interest in education was keenly expressed from one generation to the next.

The earliest Beach transplant, John ("The Pilgrim") Beach (1620-1681) was said to have been born in Devon, England in 1620. Beach and his brothers, Richard and Thomas, were among the first English settlers of New Haven, Connecticut. John became a landowner, a critical measure of a man's success. He and his wife Mary, whom sources claim was "a Danish lady," lived in Stratford with their ten children.[7] John Beach was made the local auctioneer and "Crier for the town" and "allowed four pence for everything he cries."[8]

The Beachs' fourth son, Isaac (1669-1741), married Hannah Birdsey, the daughter of a wealthy settler. Descendants recall that he was a successful tailor and that he and Hannah raised a family of six, including a son John (1700-1782) who became a well-known local minister. He and his first wife Sarah raised a large family and their fourth son, Lazarus, was Walter Ladd's paternal great-great-grandfather.[9]

Lazarus Beach, Sr. inherited a significant amount of land from his father and this made it possible for him to play a prominent role in public affairs in the towns of Newtown and Redding. He was well remembered as an advocate for local education, a value he passed forward to his son, Lazarus Beach, Jr. who was a man of many talents—a printer, bookseller, and publisher of broadsides and periodicals including Bridgeport, Connecticut's first newspaper, the *American Telegraph and Fairfield County Gazette*. The *Gazette*, which circulated over 800 copies, was founded in 1795 and delivered weekly by post-rider throughout Fairfield County at a subscription rate of $1.50 annually.[10]

Kate hoped that her mother would be impressed to learn that Walter's great-grandfather Beach was "an intimate" of the Marquis de Lafayette. An indication of their friendship was a green baize chair and desk that the Marquis presented to him. These were the very furnishings upon which the general once sat to write letters and take tea. Kate planned to emphasize that the American Beach line America was founded in 1643, preceding her mother's Everit line.

Walter's ancestor Lazarus married Polly Thompson Hall in 1797 at Trinity Church in Southport, Connecticut. She was a young widow with several children from her first marriage to Dr. Charles Hall. Her family could also boast of strong American roots. Thompson was a common name among the early settlers of New England, most of whom had emigrated from London or Hertfordshire. Polly's antecedent, Anthony Thompson and his wife, children and brothers were among a group that set sail from England on the *Hector* arriving at Boston in the summer of 1637. The Thompsons, dissenters from the Church of England like the Macys, secured agricultural land in New Haven and subsequent generations remained in the area. Polly's father and Walter's great-great-grandfather, Hezekial Thompson apprenticed as a saddler but ultimately studied the law and commenced the practice of this profession at Woodbury, Connecticut. He also served in the army at Fort William Henry near Lake George, New York during the French and Indian War. At home in Woodbury, he and his wife Rebecca raised a large family. He was a man of local prominence, a magistrate, Justice of the Peace, and a representative to the General Assembly. Like the Beaches, Thompson placed a high value on education; three of his sons were college graduates.[11]

Early in his marriage, Lazarus Beach departed from his typical subject matter, which was aimed at a male readership and initiated a new venture. In 1798 he advertised a new journal "calculated entirely for the ladies" and called it *The Hummingbird or Herald of Taste*. The journal's inaugural issue, published April 14, 1798, offered an address to the "Patrons of the Hummingbird" in all likelihood penned by a woman editor, possibly his wife Polly. It read,

> I know it will be argued that it is a woman's business to attend to her family concerns, and that she has no business to be inquisitive about what is going forward in the world. I acknowledge that domestic affairs are her business; and this business, with industry she may conduct properly, and have much time to read. I will not neglect my spinning wheel, even to compile the *Humming Bird*, for I think you had better be without

entertainment, than my children without clothes.[12]

The journal's "female editor" continued with the promise that "the news which will be published in the Paper will only be of a Domestic Kind, and as such concerns ladies only. Political and commercial details will be excluded." She emphasized her desire to solicit articles from other ladies but hoped to secure contributions from "literary gentlemen" as well.[13] Sadly, the *Hummingbird* was but a fleeting publication. However, if Polly Beach did in fact serve as the journal's female editor, the short life of the journal may be easily explained. In November of 1798, seven months after the *Hummingbird's* initial appearance, Polly gave birth to a stillborn son. She went on to bear three daughters. The first was Fanny, born in 1800 and named after one of Polly's daughters from her first marriage. The family moved to New York City and in about 1802 Beach established an office at 358 Pearl Street where he began to publish the *New-York Journal Weekly Monitor* with Samuel Mallory. This endeavor and several later attempts at newspaper publishing failed over the course of the next five years.[14] Nevertheless, the Beaches remained in New York where Lazarus died in 1816. Two years later Fanny married James Ladd; by the early 1820s they were well acquainted with William Whitehead for whom they named Walter's father.

The Ladd-Whitehead arrangement was somewhat out of the ordinary. If Charles Dickens had set one of his novels in New York, it might have been a tale about a kind Scottish benefactor devoted to a growing American family, a well-off man who provides the head of the household with employment as well as a home for his wife and children. In return his needs are attended to by his employee's wife— she prepares his meals, mends his clothes and maintains his rooms, all while caring for her husband and sons and daughters in sickness and in health. James, Fanny, and their offspring became William Whitehead's family. Their lives were played out in close quarters; perhaps the merchant and Fanny Beach Ladd were intimately drawn to each other while Fanny was still a young woman. This would help to explain the enduring nature of their association. One Ladd descendent has suggested that William and Fanny were lovers and that Whitehead fathered at least some of the Ladd children.[15]

Kate was intrigued by the Scottish merchant who, like the Macys, conducted business in New York and she wanted her mother to know that Walter's step-grandfather was a charitable man of means. He was a member of the Scottish St. Andrew's Society which had been founded in part "to provide relief of natives of Scotland and their descendants who may be in want or distress, to provide educational assistance to natives of Scotland and their descendants, to conduct and sponsor such other and further activities, as may be deemed appropriate or desirable by the Society..."[16]

According to the Society's Annals,

> William Whitehead, son of John Whitehead and Margaret Wingate, was born at Touch, Parish of St. Ninian's, Stirling, Dec. 17, 1786. In 1825 we find him engaged in business, believed to be importing, at 83 Pine St. He migrated back and forth between Pine and Cedar Streets up to 1844 when he seems to have retired from business and moved to Throgg's Neck, Westchester County. In 1845 Mr. Whitehead was rated at $150,000. He married at Throgg's Neck, Mrs. Fanny B. Ladd, a widow with two sons and three daughters. Mr. Whitehead died at Throgg's Neck, May 22, 1866. His property was left to his widow for life and the reversion to her children. The widow died in Brooklyn, March 14, 1868.[17]

William Whitehead paid $25,000 for an estate of about sixty acres in Westchester County in November 1843.[18] Joining William Whitehead at Throggs Neck shortly thereafter were James Ladd, who would manage the estate, his wife Fanny, and four children. Their three-year-old daughter, Fanny Beach, had recently died, and at the age of forty-two, Fanny Ladd was again heavy with child. A daughter Catherine was born at Throggs Neck in June. It is difficult to imagine how Fanny Ladd felt about leaving her home at 114 Sixteenth Street, in the midst of the city, for a place as distant as Throggs Neck where she faced an isolated existence. Like many women of modest means, Walter's grandmother's married life was fraught with difficulty due to her frequent pregnancies. She gave birth to twelve children including a set of twins, over the course of twenty-five years. Coping with so many pregnancies as well as the demands of childrearing, nursing sickly offspring, and tending to two adult men must have taken a toll. Seven of the dozen Ladd children died before reaching their third birthday and Fanny learned firsthand that even seemingly healthy adult children could be taken in the blink of an eye. Her oldest child,

Fanny Sophia, the new bride of a Scottish doctor, was struck down at the age of nineteen.

Whatever foreboding she might have felt initially, over time Fanny discovered that the move to Throggs Neck signaled a positive change for her. Despite the more isolated nature of country life, she was joined by two women who helped to alleviate her household burdens. They were Sarah Hannan Phillips who married Walter's father in 1851 and Maria Utter (alternatively spelled Otter or Otto) who maintained long-term ties with the family, living with Walter's aunt Ellen Ladd Wallace once she moved to Brooklyn. In addition to being able to enjoy regular female companionship, Fanny came to appreciate that living conditions on a country estate in the mid-nineteenth century were more salubrious than those found in the close quarters of the city where disease was always at the ready to snatch away life. At Throggs Neck, fresh air and wholesome food were abundant, allowing her children and grandchildren to thrive. Sadly, her husband was not so fortunate. He died eight years after he had begun farming in what was then Westchester County.[19] Two years later, Fanny and William Whitehead wed; they spent a dozen years together as man and wife and Whitehead was the only grandfather the Ladd boys, who were raised on his sixty-acre estate, ever knew. He died in 1866 and was buried in vault 176 at the New York City Marble Cemetery on Second Street; Fanny and other Ladd family members were interred in the vault as well. After Fanny died Walter's father and siblings sold the Throggs Neck land, house, and outbuildings to sugar refiner Frederick C. Havemeyer, Jr. for $100,000, (more than $1.7 million dollars in today's money) which left Walter's parents comfortably well-off for the first time in their lives.

Kate may have found the complex web of Walter's ancestral narrative family line somewhat bewildering. Her ability to comprehend her own lineage was facilitated by a reliance on her Uncle Silvanus's extensive Macy genealogy book as well as regular conversation with family members. She was accustomed to straightforward familial relationships and she had never encountered a couple who lived with a "benefactor." All of this made Walter seem even more mysterious and appealing.

Chapter 10

KATE WAS QUICKLY INFATUATED BY WALTER LADD. He paid her more attention than anyone ever had with the exception of her father, and she was captivated by his charm and maturity. Nevertheless, she knew that her mother would be alarmed by her interest in an "older man" especially one who had no connection to the Macys or their society. Therefore, when Kate initially spoke to her mother about Walter she simply described him as one of her new Richfield companions. This conversation occurred shortly before the Macys' planned departure from Richfield Springs; they were finishing off their summer holiday with a stay at Blue Mountain Lake in the Adirondacks. Kate was desperate to continue to spend time with Walter. Even though they had been acquainted for less than two weeks, she convinced her mother to allow her to invite him and two of his chums, Louis DuBois and John Seely Ward to join them on the next leg of their holiday.

In 1881 the trip to Blue Mountain Lake was an arduous one; Kate and her party journeyed through miles of virgin wilderness by train and buckboard. Once there, they met with other friends and relatives including Amelia Willets, one of Carrie's dearest friends and a fellow member of the Society of Friends. Amelia's son Howard, who was exactly two years older than Kate, was considered to be a future match for her.

Throughout their stay in the mountains, Carrie treated Walter cordially, believing that Kate viewed him as nothing more than a summer friend. However, this was not the case: On their final day in Richfield Springs Walter met with Kate privately and told her that he cared for her. Kate was thrilled at the prospect of having Walter as a suitor, but she kept the true nature of their relationship to herself. Once she returned home, however, Kate intended to continue to keep company with her new beau. She knew that the time had come to disclose the true nature of her feelings toward Walter Ladd to her mother. Kate recalled years later, "After a few weeks' acquaintance,

Walter Ladd wanted to marry me, which put my poor mother in a state of despair as she felt I was too young to think of marriage."[1]

Carrie was alarmed by her daughter's revelation and she was adamantly against Kate keeping company with "Mr. Ladd." Even though Kate felt certain that Walter was an honorable man from a good family, her mother was skeptical about his true intentions toward her daughter; the daughters of affluent men were expected to marry within their class. In Carrie's mind, it was also important that a potential mate have a similar religious background as well as a business connection, someone like Howard Willets. As far as she was concerned Walter Ladd was completely unsuitable for Kate. Not only did she believe that Walter was too old for Kate—he was twenty-five—Carrie was concerned that he lacked ambition and family connections. Although Walter was employed as a clerk in a commission business and had recently been involved with the importation of grapes from Malaga, Spain, Carrie reminded Kate that at his age her father, Josiah, was considered a leading light in the oil industry. It was no secret that Kate's mother feared that Walter was more interested in the Macy fortune than in Kate, and she suggested that this might have been why he seemed to show an interest in Mae during the first few days at Richfield Springs. In other words, any Macy daughter would do.

Carrie's words stung Kate but did not dissuade her from keeping company with Walter. She had a history of willful behavior; she had been adept at manipulating her father who often served as a buffer between mother and daughter and she was determined to defy her mother as she continued to encourage Walter's attentions. To Carrie's dismay, in September 1881, less than two months after they first met, Walter left his parents' home in Brooklyn for good and took a room in Forty-Seventh Street to be close to Kate and spend all of his free time with her. This put Carrie Macy into a particularly difficult situation; she desperately wanted to pry her daughter away from Walter Ladd. Alone as a widow, she felt ill-equipped to protect Kate from "outsiders" with questionable motives—this was a father's duty. As she fretted over the situation, she keenly felt her husband's absence, believing that if he were alive, he, too, would fear for Kate's well-being and support her position. Despite her mother's unease Kate was delighted with her suitor and especially happy to have him living nearby.

Carrie's concern for her daughter was legitimate; Kate truly was young and inexperienced, and Walter Ladd had pursued her with lightning speed. Carrie was troubled further that the Ladds were unknown to her large circle in Brooklyn. Had Kate's uncles made discreet inquiries about the object of their niece's affections, they would have corroborated that Walter worked downtown as a clerk in the fruit importation business. In addition, they would have told Carrie that prior to meeting Kate, Walter was known to hob-nob in Brooklyn where he attended parties and weddings, joined the local boating club, and pursued the gay life of the yachting set. Carrie concluded that Walter was from a better-than-average family and that he had been raised in the shadow of refinement thanks to his step-grandfather William Whitehead. Nonetheless, she speculated that this might have left him with a taste for the finer things in life.

Despite her family's unease, Kate was convinced that Walter loved her. She was thrilled that with a room on Forty-Seventh Street they could meet on every occasion including on Sundays for a walk after church. Walter managed to become acquainted with all of Kate's friends, and he was asked to all the fashionable dances.[2] Carrie, however, remained wary of Walter's motivations: Was he determined to accompany her daughter about town because he cared for her, as Kate believed, or did he escort her about for his personal social advancement? More than a century later a Macy descendant echoed the sentiment that spanned later generations when she said, "Everyone in the family has always said that Kate Macy made an inappropriate marriage."[3]

As the fall progressed, Carrie found her daughter's romance to be more than she could handle and, unexpectedly, in the midst of the social whirl of Kate's coming-out year she decided "to carry the family off to Lakewood" in New Jersey where they "spent a dreary month" with Carrie reading George Eliot's *Middlemarch* to her girls.[4] The Macys went to the newly christened town of Lakewood to keep Kate and Walter apart. Ultimately, Carrie's plan backfired.

Since Lakewood was an easy train trip from New York City and was known to have a somewhat milder climate, the town was promoted as a convenient winter playground for New Yorkers. The Macys took rooms at the Laurel House Hotel. Kate viewed this interlude as her punishment and her mother's attempt to dictate how she should conduct her life. Carrie hoped that her daughter would forget Walter in the elegant comfort of the hotel where dances and outdoor excursions for the younger set were scheduled daily. Nevertheless, Kate refused to participate and showed no interest in meeting the eligible young men who were also on holiday. Instead, she passed her time indoors longing for Walter; she described the month at Lakewood as "a month never to be forgotten."[5] She was not permitted to see or hear from Walter, and exhibiting her willfulness, she stopped eating. She grew so thin that her mother became worried and moved the family back to New York where Walter was sent word that he could visit her. Carrie said to Kate, "We will say nothing about an engagement for the time being," to which Kate defiantly replied, "We are engaged now." Carrie emphasized that it was premature to think about an engagement, and she reminded her daughter that she had known Walter for but a few months. Kate told her mother that while she would never marry without her consent, she would never marry anyone but Walter Ladd.[6]

On February 4, 1882, six months after they had met at the Richfield Springs dance, and two months shy of Kate's nineteenth birthday the couple formally announced their engagement, but no immediate wedding date was set.[7] As a mature woman Kate recalled these months with a touch of sadness, admitting that while she and Walter had "a hard time" she believed that her mother suffered even more.[8]

Carrie's plan to break up her daughter's liaison had failed miserably. Nevertheless, she was so uncomfortable about the engagement that she continued to seek ways to put distance between Walter and Kate. She abruptly announced that she and her children would be traveling abroad with Mary and William Kingsland and that Kate's former teacher, Julia Nott, would join them. Carrie hoped that a long and stimulating travel experience with opportunities to meet men whom she considered to be more socially suitable would cause Kate to forget Walter once and for all. One can imagine the gloomy scene at the Macy house as Kate absorbed the news and conveyed it to her fiancé. Despite her unhappiness over the plans for the "Grand Tour" of Europe, Kate acquiesced to her mother's wishes, knowing that she would find a way to see Walter while abroad. The family sailed on the *Alaska* on April 25, 1882, and although it was considered to be the fastest ship of the day, the voyage seemed endless. Kate recalled the day she set sail as "a sad day for Walter and I."[9] The crossing was rough but the thought of a six-month separation was even more unbearable.

Although Kate initially undertook the journey in a state of misery she came to appreciate many aspects of her first trip to Europe and kept a travel diary to record the details of her experience. After a week at sea the *Alaska* reached the port of Liverpool, "a most unattractive place, where we spent only one night."[10] The party moved on to London and spent several weeks touring in and around the city, thanks to the efforts of Miss Nott and William Kingsland whom Kate considered to be delightful travelers. The pair did all the planning; they were keen for the Macys to see every well-known place of interest and Kate seemed keen to absorb it all. She wrote in her memoir,

We had unusually good weather for London, and many pleasant drives and walks in Hyde Park. The hansoms fascinated me, also the four-in-hand coaches on which we took many excursions to places of interest in the vicinity of London. After two weeks in that interesting city, we proceeded to Leamington, Stratford-on-Avon, and Warwick. I well remember the picturesque castles of the latter place. Our next visit was to the charming ruins of Melrose and Dryurgh Abbey and on up through the beautiful English Lakes district, stopping on our way to see our first impressive Cathedral at York. We arrived just in time for late afternoon service and I have never since heard such a lovely boy's voice; it rang out in the old Cathedral like a beautiful clear bell, and almost seemed like a voice from another world... We also visited the Scotch Lakes. Scotland never impressed me as a place I wanted to live in; the hills are so bare, although the yellow gorse is very beautiful...We left the British Isles with regret...[11]

The family's tour took them to the continent—to Brussels, the Hague, and Amsterdam, but it was Paris that captivated Kate. No doubt she had yearned to see the city where her sister had enjoyed herself with abandon when she accompanied the Kingslands there after their father died. Kate described the city as "...my beloved Paris—no place on earth quite like it, where one's eyes feast on beauty at every turn..." She further praised Venice and wrote of arriving there, "one lovely moonlight night when we all felt we had reached fairyland...we wondered when the people slept for we were kept awake all night by beautiful singing under our windows; so fascinating, we were willing to go without sleep..."[12]

William Kingsland and Miss Nott, who presumably served as the Macy girls' chaperone, kept their party moving at a feverish pace throughout the spring and early summer. It appears that Kate was happy and distracted by the excitement of all that she encountered and this soothed her mother to a great degree. However, unbeknownst to Carrie, she had been kept in the dark: Kate and Walter maintained a furtive transatlantic correspondence, and they made plans to meet in Europe. In Kate's mind fortune came to her rescue when Walter wrote that a junior partner, who was residing in Spain, was taken ill with typhoid fever. As a result, he said that he was obliged to travel to Malaga to relieve him, and once the man recovered Walter arranged to go home by way of the Continent, enabling him to spend two weeks with the Macys in Switzerland that August.

It is easy to imagine that heated conversation ensued when Kate divulged that she and Walter were to be reunited. Carrie was incensed to learn that the couple's romance had thrived and that her daughter's enjoyment of the trip had not diminished her longing for Walter as she was led to believe. In all likelihood Kate's mother questioned whether "fortune" had rescued Kate and Walter, or if they had secretly plotted their reunion, fabricating the ruse of a sick partner in Malaga. Nonetheless, by the end of his visit in Switzerland, Carrie realized that she had been beaten and that her daughter would only marry Walter Ladd. Although she accepted Kate's demand, she never fully accepted Walter as a son-in-law, even though throughout the rest of her lifetime he behaved as a model husband. He always tried to ingratiate himself with his mother-in-law so that Kate could feel that her mother had been wrong about him.

Walter returned to New York on the *Germanic* and Kate joined him at home in mid-October after five full months of travel. While she was in Europe Walter's father, William Whitehead Ladd had twice called upon her grandfather but William Macy, Sr. commented that he was not enthusiastic about becoming acquainted with the Ladds. Like Carrie, Kate's grandfather and uncles were disappointed in her choice of husband; they viewed Walter as a working man devoid of means or an inheritance of any consequence. Although he may have applied himself to his work, the Macys did not consider him to be a man moving up in life. In the end, however, they did not stand in the couple's way; they adopted a veneer of civility toward the Ladds as was characteristic of their station, and Kate jubilantly began to plan her wedding.

After her peripatetic months abroad, Kate gratefully settled back into everyday life in New York. Her evenings were reserved for Walter, who was dutifully occupied at his downtown office throughout the week. Winter and spring passed pleasantly with events such as dances, dinners, and receptions. Kate proudly introduced her fiancé to congregants at the Fifth Avenue Church, and Walter became better acquainted with the Reverend Dr. Hall. After church the young people frequently traveled to Brooklyn to pass a quiet Sunday with the Ladds at their brownstone on President Street.

While her evenings and weekends were reserved for Walter, during the week Kate enjoyed spending time with her fun-loving group of female friends, many of whom she had known since girlhood. Following their coming-out year, the young women hatched a plan for a "club," which after some deliberation they decided to call "Meet Every Five" or M.E.F. They agreed that their lives were all changing so quickly that it was impossible to know what the future might bring. Kate and her friends made a pact that no matter where life might take them they would meet for a reunion in New York City every five years so that they would never drift apart.

Chapter 11

KATE RELISHED TWO TANGIBLE SYMBOLS of her hard-won engagement—a dainty sapphire and diamond ring and an extravagant, hand-pieced engagement quilt. The ring was a daily reminder of Walter's affection; the quilt signified that her engagement to Walter was incontrovertible. The luxurious bedcover was based on a design of interlocking silk hexagons of both dull and shiny or satin texture, which were joined together to form the cover and backed with a rich, wine-colored silk satin. Uniform paper hexagons were then covered with cloth, the edges carefully folded over and basted to secure them. Two of these were placed face to face, and one side of the hexagon was carefully whipstitched. Other pieces were added using the same method. It was a tried and true pattern with roots in the 1830s, when it had been popularized in England; it was alternately called "Mosaic," "Hexagon," or "Honeycomb." The design instructions were first published in the fashionable *Godey's Lady's Book* in January 1835.[1] The quilt, which was known to be difficult to piece due to its intricacy, was created by the hands of Kate's female friends and relatives representing both the Macy and Ladd sides of the family.

Kate's engagement quilt is covered with more than one hundred interlocking floral clusters which when viewed from a distance, are mesmerizingly kaleidoscopic. Upon close inspection the pattern brings to mind a flower garden with colors both bright and muted. Each posy in the patch flaunts an intricate or whimsical embroidered detail at its center, elaborate monograms and pet and family names such as "Sallie" and "Nannie," "Auntie," "Mama," and "Sister." There are also pictures, delicately rendered in thread: a wise owl, Asian inspired lanterns and fans, floral bouquets, sheaves of wheat, and quite interestingly, a charming "Kate Greenaway" girl based upon an illustration from the 1879 bestselling children's book, *Under the Window*. Randomly placed throughout the quilt top are patches embroidered with the letters "M.E.F." in recognition of Kate's friends and their commitment to meet every five years. Anchoring the design is the quilt's large central medallion, a field of wine satin where pink posies bloom. Kate's maiden initials "K.E.M." are encircled by delicate buds, leaves, and vines. The quilt is a tender representation of women's imagination working together to bring a lifetime of love and good wishes for the future Mrs. Walter Ladd.

The Macy women were especially occupied with their embroidery hoops that winter. Kate's first cousin Eliza, one of Uncle Silvanus's daughters, was also engaged. Her fiancé was the girls' cousin Silvanus Folger Jenkins, who was at one time considered a potential match for Kate's sister Mae. Kate was sensitive about her sister's feelings; she knew that by custom, as the older sister, Mae should have been the first to receive an engagement ring and quilt and walk down the aisle in a cloud of white. With her wedding date set for December 5, 1883, she chose Mae to be her bridesmaid.

Carrie Macy and the Kingslands leased a large, shingle-style house called Cleftstone at Bar Harbor, Maine, the summer before Kate's wedding. The attractive home was designed by architect Bruce Price, known for building the Hotel Frontenac in Quebec City, and it had six bedrooms and a separate dwelling for staff.

Bar Harbor appealed to Carrie since the town was less ostentatious than the more popular summer resort of Newport. Despite her wealth and admiration of finery, she remained very much an unpretentious Quaker at heart. Nonetheless, by 1883, Bar Harbor was in the throes of a transformation. Although older hotels such as the Agamont House, The Rodick, and The Rockaway continued to attract summer guests, a new breed of visitor had begun to show the desire and capacity to build distinctive private residences. Opulent dwellings designed by prominent architects wishing to show off their talent were rising up on the outskirts of the compact commercial village center. These commissions featured romantic turrets, towers, and balconies placed to capitalize on outstanding water views. The houses were quaintly referred to as "cottages" despite their substantial size and cost and their affluent owners became the talk of the town. The locals, awed by the newcomers' riches, expected to benefit from this unexpected incursion of wealth.

Indicative of the changes afoot, a correspondent for the *Mount Desert Herald* noted that Bar Harbor was "settling into a quiet elegance." Rustic calico dresses were being replaced with fashionable summer gowns for daytime and evening wear, and "High teas, dinner parties and all sorts of excursions left no idle moment."[2] Another writer editorialized that cottage life was becoming distinct from hotel life and that cottagers were providing their own forms of entertainment including musicales, suppers, and dances. The younger set preferred dances and parties over more rustic outdoor activities, and some feared that Bar Harbor was on its way to becoming a stylish watering-hole like Newport, Long Branch, and Saratoga.[3]

Kate and her mother spent hours discussing wedding plans and making social calls. These were the days before the creation of such bastions of the well-to-do as the Bar Harbor Swimming Club, the Casino, the Kebo Valley Club, and Guy Lowell's classically designed Building of Arts where Kate would one day enjoy entertainments on par with those available in New York City. When Walter visited for his two-week summer holiday, the young couple would have hired a private buckboard to take them to Schooner Head, Otter Cliffs, and Eagle Lake for a picnic and a stroll. Enterprising drivers charged summer visitors a steep rate for the pleasure of being chauffeured about in a genuine "Bar Harbor Buckboard" created by the enterprising Davis brothers, who eventually produced long wagons with rubber tires at their sizable factory on School Street in Bar Harbor. Each wagon could convey up to seventeen passengers and lent an air of frivolity to the experience of carefree holiday makers. [4]

It was at Bar Harbor that Kate's mother became better acquainted with Mrs. Miles Buck Carpenter, whom she knew from her neighborhood in New York City as well as through Kate's church. Josephine James Carpenter was a charming woman. The daughter of a housepainter, scandal mongers hinted that her heritage was Dutch and possibly Hebrew on her mother's side. No one was certain, but they whispered that her perennially absent husband, Miles Buck Carpenter, was a philanderer who had accumulated a fortune through a variety of suspect enterprises. Carrie Macy did not care for gossip. It was enough for her to know that Miles Carpenter was raised by a New York Quaker mother and might be distantly related to the Macys to make her silence anyone who wished to engage in idle talk about her friend.

Once the Macys resumed residence on Fifty-Third Street, Kate focused on her wedding preparations. Like many brides of her era Kate chose a white wedding gown, a tradition popularized by Queen Victoria who wore white when she married Prince Albert in 1840.

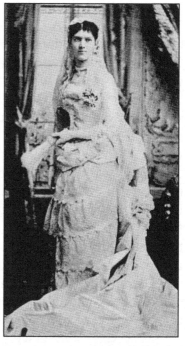

Prior to this woman were known to be wed in dresses of any fashionable hue. Taking a cue from the Queen, ladies magazines promoted the color white for wedding dresses through advice columns and printed fashion-plates: "Fashion has dictated, from the earliest ages, that white is the most fitting hue, whatever may be the material. It is an emblem of purity and innocence of girlhood, and the unsullied heart she now yields to the chosen one."[5]

Given her family's wealth Kate would have been provided with an extensive trousseau. It included carefully wrapped chemises, trimmed in lace, nightdresses, drawers, embroidered camisoles, silk and cashmere vests, French corsets and corset covers, brocade petticoats, satin dressing gowns, dainty hankies, and silk stockings. To prepare her for

Kate's wedding portrait, age 20 *(Courtesy of the Macy Family)*

married life seamstresses sewed walking dresses, traveling dresses, and velvet and silk day and evening frocks, which were accessorized with multiple hats, pairs of shoes, muffs, parasols, and pairs of gloves. Etiquette books advised brides-to-be to furnish a wardrobe for "at least two years, in underclothes, and one year in dresses, though the bonnet and cloak suitable for the coming season are all that are necessary, as the fashions in these articles changes so rapidly."[6]

The Macy-Ladd nuptials took place on a Wednesday evening. Perhaps Kate chose to marry in mid-week based on the promise of the words of a popular rhyme:

Marry on Monday for health,

Tuesday for wealth,
Wednesday is the best day of all,
Thursday for crosses, Friday for losses,
And Saturday for no luck at all.

It stands to reason that Carrie Macy faced her daughter's wedding day with a mixture of emotion. Kate's decision to marry Walter Ladd had caused tremendous friction between mother and daughter, and Carrie was not convinced that her child had chosen her husband wisely. Her outlook was further tinged with sadness because Kate's wedding day fell just a few days before Carrie's forty-fifth birthday and what should have been her silver wedding anniversary. She missed her husband, and it must have been heartrending for her to witness their daughter's marriage without him, especially when the ceremony was performed by a Presbyterian minister. Dr. Hall's involvement reminded Carrie that the comforting traditions of the Religious Society of Friends with which she had been raised were fading. This was underscored by the fact that Kate's official resignation from the New York Monthly Meeting was recorded as the date of her marriage, December 5, 1883.

Despite the fact that Kate's mother may have been in a wistful mood, a peek into the Macy parlor on the evening of December fifth offers a scene of opulence and happy contentment. With the help of her sister Mae, Kate gracefully descends the staircase. She is tightly corseted and clutches an ivory fan; her gown exudes high fashion and good taste and she is the picture of purity from head to toe, her face concealed by an exquisite rose point lace veil. Perhaps Kate lingers a bit on those familiar stairs, knowing that she has left behind her old familiar life, much of it spent with Mae in their girlhood bedroom. The strains of an organ drift in the background and a large assemblage of guests wait below with the anxious groom and the Reverend Dr. Hall. The bride steps into the candlelit parlor and the wedding ceremony gets underway.

Nonetheless, Kate offers scant detail about her wedding,

On December 5th we were married in my home, No. 18 West Fifty-Third Street by Dr. Hall at seven-thirty in the evening. A large reception followed, it being a gloriously clear night. The house, although large was packed and some people were afraid the stairs would give way. We left at ten-thirty and spent the night at the Windsor Hotel, Fifth Avenue and Forty-Sixth and Forty-Seventh Streets, which has since been destroyed by fire.[7]

Two days later a brief wedding announcement appeared in a Brooklyn newspaper.

Married

Ladd-Macy Wednesday evening, December 5, 1883 at the residence of the bride's mother by the Rev. John Hall, DD. Walter Graeme Ladd and Kate Everit Macy.[8]

Fortunately, Kate's aunt Mary Kingsland's diary entry offers an additional glimpse.

My dear little niece Kate married Walter Ladd last evening-They both are so happy in each other that I trust a happy life together may be in store for them. They are both Christians and try to live up to what they think is right, so their commencement in life will I trust be sanctified by God's blessing—and they may continually walk in his ways.

By 1883, the honeymoon was no longer an occasion for a bride and groom to travel with their parents as Carrie and Josiah had done twenty-five years before. Affluent young women anticipated honeymoons in romantic locales for extended periods of time. However, this was not the case for Kate, who had married a working man. Her honeymoon was a combination of one night in a New York hotel followed by a trip to Philadelphia to visit Walter's younger brother.

Three hours after Kate took her wedding vows she was whisked off to the Windsor Hotel. The place lacked intimacy (the building swallowed up an entire city block) but it was one of the city's most fashionable locales. The Windsor was known to host heads of state, like her father's Centennial year acquaintance Emperor Dom Pedro and American Presidents Chester A. Arthur and William McKinley as well as prominent members of New York society, many of whom maintained smart apartments there. Since the Ladds were guests for less than twenty-four hours, they would have missed the hotel's celebrated amenities such as the fine cuisine served in an elegant dining room where frescoes and shimmering chandeliers were meant to emulate the grandeur of an Italian palazzo. Less than twelve hours after they checked in, signing the guest register as Mr. and Mrs. Walter G. Ladd for the first time, they were on their way to Philadelphia to visit James B. Ladd, who had recently launched his career as a civil engineer. Like Walter's brothers William and Henry, Jim was a well-educated and serious young man, but as most women would attest not nearly as handsome as Walter.

Although Kate may have wished for a more romantic and secluded honeymoon, she took the trip to Philadelphia in stride. Perhaps she anticipated a return to the Windsor one day, to more fully enjoy the opulence she had missed with her quick stay, but this did not come to pass. As Kate mentioned in her memoir, the Windsor was destroyed. A fire broke out one St. Patrick's Day, while thousands of New Yorkers made merry at the annual Irish parade on Fifth Avenue, after a careless hotel guest tossed a burning match in an upstairs hallway. Window drapes were ignited and rather than alert anyone, the cowardly man ran into the street to blend in with the noisy crowd. The fire quickly escalated into an inferno, trapping scores of guests and employees inside the building and transforming the happy street scene into one of horror—panic-stricken men and women screamed for help or jumped to their deaths from windows high above the sidewalk. Within an hour most of the Windsor Hotel had collapsed: In all ninety souls were lost. As she learned about this disaster Kate felt that she could easily relate to the plight of those involved having spent an important night in her life in that very place.

Upon returning from Philadelphia Kate read the congratulatory cards and letters she and Walter had received from her family. An envelope from her Aunt Carrie Lansing Everit (her mother's sister-in-law) contained two letters that Kate treasured throughout her life.

Dear Kate & Walter

In looking over recently, some letters long treasured because of association with Uncle Thomas & my early life as "Bride & Groom" was one from Kate's father: a letter so affectionate, expressing so true an interest in our welfare, at a time when entering upon a new & untried life that it has been held sacred all these twenty-one years.

The advice your father gave, & the life he lived, exemplified all he said, & as you know dear Kate his life was as nearly perfect as one can be in this world.

This letter has also been the rule of our life & now today I commend it to you both, such as touches upon your new relations-your father's own words. I am confident he would say much the same to you, were he with you this memorable day. I am sure he could say no more, as he has given the rule complete, for solid, true, happiness.

On your return Walter I shall ask you to kindly return Josiah's letter to me. I find I cling to it as something specially ours & cannot relinquish ownership even to Kate much as I should like to do so-

And now, I will only add, that my own prayer, uttered by a loving affection for you both, is that you may be blessed with many, very many years to each other, & reap, in the future, the full reward of a pure unselfish love one to the other.

With love
Aunt Carrie L Everit
142 St James Place Bklyn
Wed. Dec. 5th 1883

Kate may have felt that her deceased father spoke to her from heaven when she opened the second letter which he had written to his brother-in-law Thomas Everit when he married Carrie Lansing in 1862.

Dear Brother:

Thee has now a partner in all thy joys and all thy sorrows, one who will cherish every kind word & act. Let not a word or action of thine be the cause of one unhappy moment to her. She has forsaken a good & kind Aunt who has been unto her as a Mother, a good home and kind friends, all for thee. Her future life and happiness now depend upon thee, so let the life & actions be such that she will never have occasion to look back with sorrow to the past great act of her life. A woman's life is a hard one She has many trials to pass through and it is for thee to be unto thy wife, such a kind, loving & affectionate husband, that will make all her trials, as pleasures.

Dear Brother and Sister you have now taken the most important step in life. I hope & pray that it is right. Don't expect too much one of the other, for from thus all differences arise. Move down life's voyages together train your thoughts and wishes alike and you will find life rolls on, that this is the secret of true happiness, to have but one guardian angel, to live within each other. Never allow thyself to speak an unkind word, or act an unkind act to thy Dear Carrie for it will penetrate the inmost recess of her heart, perhaps to be forgotten, but never effaced, for as a woman was made higher than man, she is capable of much deeper & stronger love than man so in like proportion her feelings are

much more easily and deeply hurt, by an unkind word from one, who she loves unto death. I write this dear Brother & Sister out of pure love & affection for you both, that your lives may be one continual sunshine.

Thy dear Sister Carrie Everit Macy has been unto me all that man could ask. She has brought me more happiness than I ever expected in this world, and I wish for her Brother, the same.

With many kind wishes for your future happiness, I am your

Bro.

J. Macy Jr.

Carrie sends her love

Josiah's poignant advice, written at age twenty-four, provides a glimpse into his tender and mature heart. Kate tucked both of the letters into the back pocket of her Bible where they remained for more than one hundred twenty-five years. Later in life, as her nieces and nephews were preparing for marriage she shared her father's advice, stressing that "one of the most important things in starting life together is not to expect too much one of the other."

Chapter 12

WHILE KATE AND WALTER WERE IN PHILADELPHIA her mother and sister Mae moved all of their wedding gifts to a "cute little" apartment at 210 West Fifty-Seventh Street so that when the newlyweds returned the apartment was is perfect order; even their first dinner awaited them. Kate commented, "I don't believe any two people ever enjoyed a little home of their own as much as we did. The apartment seemed just perfect in every way."[1]

As they settled into their new routine as husband and wife the Macy clan continued to grow. Kate and her cousins, Clara and Sallie, were all expecting babies. However, by early May Kate's pregnancy was in danger as she had developed Scarletina, which was a variation of Scarlet Fever that more commonly affected children. It was known that Scarletina could affect a woman's ability to carry a child to term.

Kate's feelings toward her mother had changed with her marriage and pregnancy, and she yearned for Carrie's comfort and care. Nevertheless, since Scarletina was highly contagious she was advised to remain in her own home. Kate recovered physically from the illness but the miscarriage that resulted left her devastated and quite possibly without the degree of understanding and support she needed. Her family felt relieved that she had recovered. On the heels of her misfortune Kate learned that a cousin had died while giving birth to her first child. Her newborn son survived and was named Clarence Macy Chauncey—Clarence after his departed mother Clara.

With the loss of her child, Kate's newfound happiness vanished into thin air. Her mother-in-law Sarah Ladd, a peaceful and spiritual woman, wrote,

> May 7th, 1884
> My dear Kate,
> I have just received your kind letter, and although I expect, and sincerely hope to be with you Early tomorrow, the weather continues so stormy, and I must send you a line tonight. How thankful I am to hear you have no pain. I cannot but be anxious,

and troubled, however, for I well know how pain has weakened
you considerably. Do be very careful for awhile yet. I cannot tell
you my darling child how my heart aches for you. I realize how
you feel, and am glad you wrote as you did—I know from
Experience how worried—how anxious you are—and my heart
full of loving sympathy is all yours.

For your Mother too—she has my warmest sympathy- I
wish I could be of some use to her. I nursed my four boys with
the fever and realize how hard it is for her to bear. What a trial of
patience and faith. So my dearie, try not to worry. Your Mother
is right in not having you go there. You would only increase her
care and add new and great risks—and your beloved husband- he
too would be inexpressibly worried. Oh, my child! It is hard I
know, but Our good Father's loving kindness will sustain you.
To His love and Mercy I must resign you and your loved ones—
that God may bless you all is my fervent prayer. With best love
to your dear self and Walter, in which Father joins, I remain your
loving Mother.

S.H. Ladd

P.S. I will be over early first clear morning—please let me
hear from you dear child, if you are not as well.

At the time of Kate's miscarriage doctors were well-aware of the
danger associated with Scarletina contracted during pregnancy.
Medical manuals asserted that there was "probably no form of
sickness which the public hold in such dread as Scarletina in
association with pregnancy…the course of pregnancy will seriously
be endangered."[2] In his series of lectures on abortion and miscarriage,
terms that were used interchangeably, noted gynecologist Dr.
Theodore Gaillard Thomas stated, "[A]mong the poisons in the blood
which are capable of causing abortion are those which create the
exanthematous eruptions of small-pox, scarletina, measles, etc…."[3]
Physician Dr. Thomas Trotter further suggested that miscarriage and
premature labor were inherently risky events that often led to nervous
disorders. Kate's Scarletina, contracted during the early stage of her
pregnancy, and the resultant miscarriage would affect her physical
and mental health for years to come.[4]

Kate spent the summer trying to recuperate. In early August she
and Walter dined with Kate's in-laws in Brooklyn before leaving
town to visit Walter's older brother William, his wife Elizabeth and

their little girl Elsie at St. Albans in upstate New York. At dinner, Sarah Ladd looked so ill that Kate insisted on delaying their holiday until she was better. A few days later, on Saturday morning, August 9, Walter's mother died of erysipelas, a form of streptococcal infection. Kate said this was " a terrible blow to us all, for she was an ideal wife and mother," and that she had never seen "a more beautiful faith than hers...her belief in prayer, her always cheerful point of view was a benediction to us all."[5] Sarah Ladd was the glue that kept her family together, and she had been a dependable and encouraging presence throughout Kate's recent ordeal; the still fragile young woman was heartbroken.

Kate's recovery was progressing slowly; distress over her mother-in-law's unexpected passing further affected her health. While visiting in Brooklyn, Walter's uncle, Dr. William Wallace, and her sister-in-law Elizabeth convinced her that she was a sick woman. Elizabeth took her to see Dr. T. Gaillard Thomas, the most noted gynecologist of the day. After a careful examination he told Kate, "I don't see how you have kept on your feet."[6] He promised nothing but said that if she would go to his sanitarium at 596 Lexington Avenue and stay for a few months time he might have some "news" about her condition. Her mother was upset. No one in the Macy family had ever spent time in a sanitarium. Carrie may have wondered if there was something amiss in her daughter's marriage that was interfering with her recovery; miscarriages were frequent occurrences. Why was Kate in need of round-the-clock professional care? Nevertheless, Kate checked in to "596" on October 18, 1864, ten months after she and Walter had married. By January Dr. Thomas could not report any improvement in Kate's condition and as she had developed a severe cough, he suggested that she spend her days at the sanitarium and her nights under her mother's care.

Kate's bout of Scarletina, miscarriage, and the gynecological issues that Dr. Thomas sought to cure mark the beginning of her chronically compromised state of health. In the early 1880s doctors such as Theodore Gaillard Thomas and his associate James B. Hunter offered services specifically for women at The Lexington Avenue Sanitarium. The private hospital advertised in medical journals in both the United States and Canada; referrals often came from well-intentioned family doctors or family members.

In answer to special inquiries we may state generally for the
benefit of our readers, that the general terms of this Institution
are: $40 per week exclusive of medical attendance payable
weekly to the matron; $22 per week for medical attendance;
operations extra. Charges determined by previous agreement. The
usual medical attendance includes two visits weekly from Dr.
Thomas, and as many as may be necessary from Dr. Hunter who
resides in the building, 596 Lexington Avenue.[7]

For upwards of forty dollars per week, a figure that covered room
and board and is the equivalent of more than $1,080 in today's
dollars, Kate lived among other affluent women, united by a desperate
quest for improved health. Without question Kate's mother covered
her medical expenses.

By 1884 Dr. Thomas was considered one the nation's foremost
gynecologists. He was one of many new medical specialists who
sought to treat women's ills after the Civil War; often these
physicians had little in the way of training or prior experience treating
women. During this era, gynecology was a fledgling medical
specialty, having but recently usurped the time-honored tradition of
women ministering to women. Dr. Thomas's views on women and
medical treatment were published in his seminal work, *A Practical
Treatise on the Diseases of Women.* Of refined women he stated, "The
customs of civilized life have depreciated her powers of endurance
and capacity for resisting disease." He attributed women's poor health
to a want of fresh air and exercise, excessive development of the
nervous system, inappropriate dress, imprudence during menstruation,
imprudence after parturition, the prevention of conception and
induction of abortion, and marriage with existing uterine disease.[8]

The doctor, who blamed women for their ill health, theorized
broadly about the vanity of "refined women." Of the desperate
wealthy women who sought treatment at his sanitarium he said:

Refined young women are too willing to be delicate, fragile
and incapable of endurance. They dread above all things the glow
and hue of health, the rotundity of beauty of muscularity, the comely shape which the great masters gave the Venus de Medici and
Venus de Milo. All these attributes are viewed as coarse and
unladylike...As a result how often do we see our matrons dreading
process of child-bearing as if it were an entirely abnormal and
destructive one...these are they who furnish employment for the

gynecologist and fill our homes with invalids and sufferers.[9]

Thomas was not interested in treating poor and working class women even when their health challenges mirrored those of their well-off counterparts. He focused his attention on "refined women" who became his bread and butter.

As one of his well-to-do clients, Kate believed in Dr. Thomas. She was unaware that even celebrated doctors such as Thomas were often grasping at straws when they diagnosed women's ailments; as a result much of their treatment had no basis in science. They were universally fixated on the womb and menstrual and uterine disorders. Knife-wielding practitioners ruled the day. Dr. Thomas and his associates, including Thomas Addis Emmet and the internationally known J. Marian Sims (often called the father of gynecology), routinely performed unwarranted hysterectomies, ovariotomies, and cliteridectomies. In that era doctors were woefully uninformed about the female reproductive system; Victorian doctors typically examined women patients through layers of clothing for the sake of propriety.

Some forty years before Kate's first experience with an exclusive gynecologist prior to being dubbed the father of the specialty and still unknown outside of Montgomery, Alabama, J. Marian Sims, a native-born South Carolinian, strove to make a name for himself by perfecting the surgical treatment of the vesico-vaginal fistula, a painful and enduring complication of childbirth. He conducted experimental operations on enslaved African women in a makeshift hospital without using any form of anesthesia. Sims was undeterred by failure and performed the surgery repeatedly on several women, one of whom endured thirty surgeries over the course of four years.[10] Sims became chief surgeon at the Women's Hospital in New York, which treated poor and middle-class women, but like his colleague Dr. Thomas he additionally operated his own lucrative private hospital for women of means. Sims was a hero in his day but in 2018, more than a century after it was erected, his statue was removed from Central Park due to public outrage over his cruel experimental practices.

Another well-known medical treatment of the period, called Battey's operation, or the surgical removal of the ovaries, was developed by Georgia physician Robert Battey. It was performed on women whose husbands deemed them unruly or disobedient or those who suffered from painful menstruation or nervousness. Women labeled as nymphomaniacs were also subject to the procedure. Most often completely healthy ovaries were excised by surgeons who had a limited understanding of female physiology. Battey first performed the ovariotomy or "female castration" in 1872. It reigned as one of the most frequently performed surgeries for women for two decades. It is unknown whether Kate's ovaries were removed while she was a patient at the Lexington Sanitarium but probably not. Even though Dr. Thomas was a known practitioner of the ovariotomy, he acknowledged that the procedure, which had no justifiable medical basis and resulted in premature menopause, was greatly overused.

By the early 1890s the Battey operation had fallen out of favor but not before physicians had followed the procedure, in part, to learn more about a woman's reproductive anatomy. Originally performed as a vaginal operation, surgeons came to favor the laparotomy, or the abdominal removal of a woman's ovaries, literally opening a new window into female reproductive organs. As astonishing as it may seem, prior to this, doctors possessed such a limited understanding of human reproduction that they did not even known when ovulation occurred.[11]

Even those women whose problems did not require surgery could be held hostage by poorly informed male specialists who insisted that all women's health issues were gynecological in nature. Female patients were habitually subjected to vaginal and rectal-vaginal exams by doctors who used rudimentary medical instruments, such as sponge tents (sponges soaked in chemicals and inserted into the vagina for as long as twenty-four hours) and an assortment of enemas infused with cod-liver oil or opium. As repugnant as this may sound to the contemporary reader, for women of Kate's day such practices may have been considered an improvement over the practice of affixing leeches to the female labia to affect a cure in previous generations.

Kate never discloses the nature of her treatment at Dr. Thomas's sanitarium. Was she in residence for ten months strictly to rest, or did she yield to the surgeon's knife? Were her days spent pleasantly chatting with other women as if they were meeting for tea or shopping along the Ladies' Mile, or were they punctuated by "medical attendance," which could include rough treatments—gut-wrenching enemas, uterine trusses, and vaginal pessaries?

One might ponder whether Kate actually preferred a cloistered life at Dr. Thomas's sanitarium where she was protected from life's difficulties including her mother's continued concerns about her husband's suitability. Throughout her stay Walter behaved as a dutiful husband; he was determined to prove to Kate's family that he was a model husband, and Kate looked forward to his visits at eight o'clock each morning and again in the evening. Perhaps she preferred this arrangement. Some women knew that the shelter of a private hospital made it possible to avoid a husband's sexual demands and, with thoughts of her cousin Clara's recent death following childbirth fresh in mind, Kate may have feared the possibility of another pregnancy despite her desire for a child of her own. Whatever their motivation may have been, women bore the details of their medical treatment silently. They held doctors on a pedestal and believed that they could make them healthy and whole. The luckiest women, like Kate, developed a network of support within the confines of the sanitarium. As time passed, this made it possible for her to recall only the best memories of those days, memories that were due to her camaraderie with other women, two of whom were destined to become her friends for life.

In her memoir Kate says, "One of my reasons for writing this history of my life is to show that in spite of much illness and some very hard experiences, someone has always come to help me at just the right moment which has given me a very strong faith and taken away all fear."[12] During her long months at the sanitarium she became acquainted with two women whom she described as the "dearest and best" friends of her life, Mrs. W.S Hill (Marie) and Mrs. W.S. Warner (Nettie).[13] The three women banded together to make the most of their situation and despite much suffering, they spent many happy hours together. Kate, Marie, and Nettie were all rundown and exhausted when they arrived at "596." Marie and Kate had recently miscarried, and Kate continued to grieve over the loss of her sympathetic and supportive mother-in-law Sarah Ladd. The circumstance that prompted Nettie's stay at "596" was far different. Although she was the mother of two healthy youngsters, she chose to be secluded within the confines of Dr. Thomas's sanitarium as she grappled with the aftermath of her husband's nefarious business dealings.

Kate and Marietta Ely Hill were like two peas in a pod, happily wed and anticipating bright futures as wives and mothers. Coincidentally, their husbands were distantly related and the men forged a friendship steeped in their ancestry and their common situation. A few years later Marie gave birth to a son, William Ely Hill, who was like a nephew to the Ladds. Will Hill became a syndicated cartoonist with a wide national following. His clever cartoons, comic strips, and books offered pointed commentaries on early twentieth century society. Kate took particular pleasure in the boy's artistic talent and professional success.

Nettie Herrick Warner and Kate had common acquaintances as members of Dr. Hall's church. By May 1884 Nettie had suffered a breakdown when her husband's involvement as a secondary player in a massive financial scandal was exposed in the press. W.S. Warner worked with the Wall Street brokerage firm of Grant & Ward, which "Buck" Grant, a son of former President U.S. Grant, and Ferdinand Ward had founded in 1880. Grant was the silent partner; he borrowed $100,000 to help launch the firm. Unbeknown to him, his slick-talking partner never put up his share. When Ward became desperate for another infusion of cash, he convinced Buck Grant's famous father, former President Ulysses S. Grant, to invest most of his personal fortune in the firm that bore his name.

The Grants were innocent concerning the nature of Ward's plan; it was in essence a Ponzi-type scheme, a practice known in the late nineteenth century as "rehypothecating."[14] Ward's game was to extract money from innocent investors and use it to create the impression that his firm was engaged in making above board loans to companies holding U.S. government contracts. Nettie Warner's husband worked behind the scenes to find wealthy investors to help finance the business. Described as "the fat hulking son of a well-known Manhattan merchant" Warner had failed in the world of business and by the early 1880s he was desperate for employment.[15] He met Ward through Buck Grant. Ward provided Warner with a rudimentary explanation of the workings of his company and indicated that huge profits awaited investors. He explained that government contracts were paid for after the satisfactory completion of a job and that this often required contractors to lay out a considerable sum of money. Therefore, they frequently needed to procure a loan to be repaid with interest. Grant and Ward stood at the ready to make such loans. In order to do so, they had to have access to substantial sources of ready cash.

On the surface, the business appeared to be a traditional loan company. However, Ferdinand Ward was greedy and unscrupulous and not one to allow the legalities of lending interfere with profit. He made it known that occasionally, due to the fast-moving nature of his business, he might not have the necessary funds on hand to make an advance. Rather than sacrifice a good transaction, he was willing to let a trusted and discreet investor in on the deal, borrowing cash from his "investor" to loan money to the contractor. Like Ward, the "investor" expected to realize a profit upon repayment of the loan. This scenario was entirely attractive to a man like Warner who was dazzled by the prospect of a big pay-out. Consequently, Nettie's husband became one of the swindlers' most dependable operatives. Through the firm's "robbing-Peter-to-pay-Paul" scheme, William Warner made easy money for a time. In 1882 he provided Ward with an initial "investment" of $15,000; thirty days later he was repaid $18,750, realizing an impressive twenty-five percent return on his investment in just one month's time. Warner's high return made it easy to bring in new investors. He received a commission for the investors he brought in, and before long Warner and Nettie were enjoying the high life. They maintained elegant residences on Fifth Avenue and in Long Branch, New Jersey, the tony seaside resort with ties to President Grant.

Despite her stylish life Nettie's world came crashing down when Ferdinand Ward's Ponzi scheme began to unravel. Grant and Ward and the Marine National Bank, from which Ferdinand Ward had borrowed heavily, both declared bankruptcy: The brokerage firm had managed to accrue liabilities in excess of sixteen million dollars. Ferdinand Ward vanished into thin air leaving his investors hanging— fortunes were lost and lives were destroyed. Within one week of the Grant and Ward collapse, mayhem erupted on Wall Street as a chain of additional businesses failed. Newspaper headlines blasted a single word, "Panic!" The subsequent financial crash was declared the worst since the panic of 1873.

Nettie Warner suffered a breakdown as a result of her husband's highly publicized role in the Grant and Ward debacle. When she was unable to face the world she sought refuge behind the doors of Dr. Thomas's sanitarium. Her husband was tried and jailed for his involvement in the affair; nevertheless in 1886 he was released from jail on a legal technicality. The Warners moved to England and neither one ever returned to the United States. In 1890 Warner suffered a fatal heart attack while traveling in France. Eventually, Kate's "596" companion Nettie married her former secretary James Herbert Masters, a Church of England clergyman. She and Kate remained in touch despite the distance in miles.

Chapter 13

As Kate was ending her stint at the sanitarium Carrie was making plans for a summer retreat. She leased the Greystone estate at Irvington-on-Hudson from businessman William S. Gurnee, who had recently built Beau Desert at Bar Harbor and had no further need for an estate in Westchester. With the Lexington Sanitarium closed for the months of July and August, Kate relocated to her mother's summer place. Greystone was an ideal location for her recuperation—the house was large and private with breathtaking views and soothing Hudson River breezes to combat the heat. In addition, the place was convenient to the city, which suited both Kate and her mother. Dependable rail service made it possible for Walter to take a train to his office in New York, and Carrie liked summering in close proximity to her elderly mother and in-laws.

Kate anticipated a peaceful summer. Nevertheless, the serenity that she yearned for was interrupted when Mae announced her engagement. Her sister's wedding plans threw the household into a frenzy and immediately absorbed all of Carrie's time and attention. Mae's fiancée was Howard Willets; their engagement news was not a tremendous surprise since it had long been assumed that a Macy daughter was destined to marry Howard. Kate's mother and her Auntie Amelia Willets had hoped for this from the time they were brides themselves.

Unlike Walter Ladd, Howard Willets was considered a perfectly suitable match for Kate's sister since the families had a great deal in common.

The two families grew to be as close as relatives through decades of shared business involvement and membership in the Religious Society of Friends. Kate's father Josiah and Howard's father John Titus were boyhood friends who "witnessed" each other's marriages as was the Friend's custom. When Josiah and Carrie moved uptown to West Fifty-Third Street, Howard's parents chose a town house right around the corner. The Macy children always addressed the Willets couple as "Auntie" and "Uncle" and Howard and his sisters Bessie and Helen were like cousins to Kate and her siblings; perhaps this is why she never considered Howard in romantic terms. Nevertheless, by 1885, Mae had no qualms about accepting Howard's proposal. She was almost age twenty-five and seemed overjoyed to accept Howard as her mate.

The family responded to the news of Mae's betrothal with joy. She wrote to share her happiness with the Kingslands, who were at Newport.

> Tuesday Evening, July 7, 1885
>
> My dear Aunt and Uncle,
>
> While Mama and Howard are sitting here beside me talking I write to tell you, the first ones, that we are engaged, and tomorrow I am going down to the city to tell Grandma and Grandpa. In a few days I will write again and tell you more about it and everything else that has been going on.
>
> We had such a nice visit from Auntie and Uncle Willets. Now I must close and go to bed for they are waiting for me. I shall long for and hope to have your congratulations among the very first. Howard says though my ring is not a "diamond of the first-water," he hopes it will do. Now I on the contrary think that it is and I am happy and thoroughly satisfied. I feel that I want it to please you also. As you know I have always been so fond of you both. Now I want to ask you please not to tell anybody for I do not want it to come out just yet.
>
> The bell has been rung for the house to be closed thus forcing me to say good night with lots of love, and many goodnight kisses from your own,
>
> Mae

Mae's letter shines a bright light on her joy. She and Carrie quickly set to work making wedding plans, setting the wedding date for January; in Carrie's mind there was no need for a long engagement. While Mae reveled in the excitement and attention she was being paid as a bride-to-be, we can imagine that Kate's heart ached as she recalled her mother's negative reaction when she announced her engagement to Walter several years earlier. Kate was envious of the time that Mae and Carrie spent together when she was craving support and understanding. Kate continued to be emotionally scarred by her miscarriage, and it was unknown if she would safely conceive again. As her loneliness welled up Kate especially missed the support and companionship of Marie and Nettie, women who understood her completely. She also missed Walter's regular companionship; she was accustomed to his daily visits and now that he traveled from Westchester to lower Manhattan, he had fewer hours to spend with his wife.

Kate was more than ready for a fresh start that autumn. Resuming their lives together, she and Walter began housekeeping at a new apartment at 155 West Fifty-Eighth Street. To her delight, her cousin George and his wife took an apartment directly opposite hers. Throughout the fall she felt first-rate; everyone commented that she had regained her color as well as her light-hearted spirit and sense of humor. As was expected, Kate fussed over her husband in the evenings, making sure that a proper meal had been prepared and that fresh flowers filled the silver vases in the dining room. As instructed by the lady's etiquette books of the day, Kate was prepared to share witty and interesting stories about her day or to read aloud letters from the days' post as he relaxed after dinner. She would have offered anecdotes about her lady friends and included updates about the women in her "Meet Every Five" club.

One chilly winter afternoon Kate hosted a memorable reunion at her apartment, and most of the members of the M.E.F. group were on hand. Her artistic friend Anna "Nannie" Paret, who liked to describe herself as "a struggling and ambitious artist," was the unofficial head of the group, the glue that held everyone together. Kate sent out handwritten invitations to their friends: Lila Alliger, Lucy Knevals, Sallie Whitcomb, Cornelia Williamson, Cornelia Redmond, Laura Shortridge, and Daisy Abbott. In preparation for their gathering, Kate carefully selected the menu and then made sure that the luncheon table was set with the delicate linens, china, and silver that were part of her treasure trove of wedding gifts. Her table was further enhanced by the unique placecards which Nannie had created for the occasion—each one was festooned with hand-painted birds and flowers and served as a keepsake for the occasion. It was good for Kate to enjoy a few hours of conversation and an exchange of gossip with old friends. Everyone felt the absence of one member, Jeanne "Daisy" Abbott. She was a new bride who had recently married a man with a somewhat notorious past, the dashing Italian Lieutenant Giovanni Bettini. Daisy's wedding was announced out of the blue and thrown together in a snap, a small and quiet affair with only close family members in attendance.

The M.E.F. friends were disappointed that Daisy had not chosen to include them, but Kate knew that Daisy had been through some difficulties of late. She was raised in New York City in the lap of luxury at the home of her maternal grandparents. As a young widow (or possibly a divorcee, no one really knew) Daisy's mother married William Lyman Pomeroy, a wealthy merchant with grown children, and within the prerequisite nine months Daisy had a baby sister, a situation she found humiliating. After all, she was preparing for her "coming out" year and her mother was pushing a pram. Her stepfather situated Daisy, her mother, and baby Aurelia Gladys at his country place in Stamford. But for Daisy life in Connecticut was isolating. She set off on "The Grand Tour," and while in Paris she met her future husband Lt. Bettini. He was already well-known among members of a certain set in New York due to a scandalous incident in his past involving a society woman and her daughter after which Bettini returned to Europe. The episode was all but forgotten until Daisy announced her impending marriage. She was determined to marry the passionate Italian and did not appear to be the least bit phased by his somewhat tarnished past.

The Ladds' new apartment was located in a complex at one of New York City's toniest addresses and was known by several names: "The Central Park Apartments," the "Navarro," or the "Spanish Flats." The edifice was called a tenement for the rich due to the large number of costly and luxurious dwellings that occupied a single city block. Despite the density, the apartments were spacious and magnificently appointed with some models having as much square footage as a three-story townhouse.

The Central Park Apartments were a prominent example of the Home Club movement, an early form of a co-operative apartment building. Individuals with similar tastes and social positions formed a joint stock company to develop an apartment complex as shareholders. Apartments cost between $15,000 and $20,000, and all residents were charged a monthly maintenance fee of $200; the considerable financial investment insured an elite clientele. Home club investors received perpetual leases in proportion to the shares held; they could either reside in their apartment or sublease it, subject to the approval of fellow shareholders. Some additional residences were owned jointly by the Home Club investors. These apartments could be leased and the income received helped to cover the cost of a variety of building expenses.

The Central Park Apartments were an imposing addition to Central Park South—eight individual structures that soared ten stories high. Each was named for a Spanish city, a nod to the developer's heritage and the source of the nickname "The Spanish Flats." On the park-side they were called the Madrid, Lisbon, Barcelona, and Cordova, and around the corner on Fifty-Eighth Street they were known as the Valencia, Tolosa, Salamanca, and Granada, which is where the Ladds lived. The entire complex was essentially Queen Ann in style, accented by turrets, gables and arches, and wisps of Moorish detail to further reflect the developer's heritage. The apartments were built from an unusual combination of granite, brownstone, Ohio stone, and Milwaukee and Philadelphia red brick. One distinctive design element was an extravagant, 300-foot long center courtyard. This private park was planted with trees, shrubs, and vibrant seasonal flowers which encircled a central fountain. It is easy to imagine Kate sitting on a bench in the courtyard catching a pleasant breeze among the trees or soaking up the warmth of the sun without ever leaving home.

The late 1880s was a competitive time for the building of luxury apartments by Central Park. The "Spanish Flats" project was the vision of developer Jose Francisco Navarro in conjunction with the architectural firm of Hubert, Pirsson And Company.

A contemporary publication, the 1887 edition of *How to Know New York City* by Sweetser and Ford, notes that the Central Park Apartments were constructed at a cost upwards of seven million dollars. The complex was located about one mile south of The Dakota, the yellow brick Germanesque chateau built by Henry Janeway Hardenbergh directly on Central Park West. A native of New Brunswick, New Jersey, Hardenbergh was well-known for his apartments, hotels, townhomes, churches, schools, and commercial buildings. His talent is well represented on the campus of his alma mater, Rutgers University. While he may be best remembered for elegant buildings such as the Dakota and the Plaza Hotel on Central Park South, Hardenbergh took on several important commissions in his home state including the construction of Natirar.

The combination of a prime location and affluent residents made Kate's address highly desirable in the 1880s. In addition, the "Flats" were known for their design innovation. In an era when indoor plumbing, heating and electricity were luxuries unavailable to the average American, the "Flats" offered all three amenities; heat and electricity were generated on the premises. A further convenience was the complex's private driveway, which sloped down to the building's basement level. This made it possible for carts and wagons to gain direct access into an underground street where they could unload deliveries without disturbing residents. The Spanish Flats were perhaps the largest apartment complex in the world in their heyday.

> Each building in the group held twelve enormous apartments, the largest of which included a twenty-three by twenty-nine foot drawing room, a fourteen by twenty-nine foot reception room, a fourteen by twenty-nine foot library, and a twenty by twenty-three foot dining room, as well as a kitchen, several pantries, and six bedrooms the smallest of which was fourteen by eighteen feet....It also included three servant rooms and three full bathrooms.[1]

Despite the apartments' spaciousness and opulence, Navarro's vision was fraught with problems from the start, and over time mounting financial problems resulted in financial losses for the shareholders. In 1926 the original complex was sold off piecemeal and subsequently demolished. Nevertheless, within a few years, the site was elegantly reborn as three new buildings were erected: the Italian-Renaissance style New York Athletic Club, the Art Deco Essex House Hotel, and the white brick Hampshire House. Navarro's Gilded Age creation was quickly forgotten, and the buildings that replaced it became emblematic of a storied stretch of Central Park South.

Chapter 14

NOT LONG AFTER THE RINGING IN OF THE NEW YEAR OF 1886 Mae and Howard Willets were married.

> An interesting wedding in the evening was that of Miss Mary K. Macy, daughter of the late Josiah Macy Jr. to Howard Willets which took place at the home of the bride's mother on West Fifty-Third-St. Both bride and bridegroom are Quakers, and the ceremony was performed in accordance with the quaint rites of that sect. The floral decorations were handsome and there were a large number of guests.[1]

The newlyweds took the 11:30 p.m. express for Sing-Sing and then traveled by carriage to Incleuberg to honeymoon on the Kingslands' opulent country estate.

In her diary Mary Kingsland wrote,

> January 20, 1886
> This is the date of my dear niece's marriage.
> 21st Last evening Howard and Mae repeated the Friends marriage ceremony which was never more earnestly said or with more faithful promises to love and cherish each other. How happy I hope they may be I have no words to express- I only can pray that God will bring them very near each other and best of all, that He may bring them both into his fold, making them his own loving children and filling their lives with such good things as He only can bestow.
>
> They have gone up to our country house Incleuberg to spend their first happy days together, and my dear husband with myself enjoy the feeling of adding to their happiness.

It is easy to imagine Kate's sense of envy over her sister's elegant Whartonesque honeymoon complete with a few discreet servants on hand to attend to the newlyweds' needs. As Howard assured the Kingslands,

> The people here take splendid care of us...last night Eliza surprised us by giving us some ice cream for dessert...We have not minded the weather much as we have been so happy

together...Although we have been together so much it is so different now and oh how much we enjoy it and the being everything to each other...Mary thanks you for your kind thoughts for our welfare and for thinking of opening the wine closet but we are splendidly taken care of and then you know I am a believer in temperance so I think sherry and claret plenty for our everyday use.[2]

In her memoir Kate made but the slightest mention of Mae's special day and incorrectly stated, "My dear sister married in 1885," the year before the wedding actually took place. If her name had not been recorded as a witness on the Willetses' Quaker marriage certificate, which was discovered in the attic of a descendant in County Cork, Ireland, in 2016, one might question whether she had been in attendance at all.

Soon after Mae's marriage Kate fell into a pattern of sporadic bouts of poor health. During the winter of 1887 she suffered from "serious stomach trouble."[3] which may have coincided with the announcement that Mae was expecting a baby. The proposed remedy was the milk diet.

During the late nineteenth and early twentieth century, a milk diet was a customary course of treatment for a broad range of illnesses including indigestion, infertility, insomnia, asthma, hay fever, rheumatoid arthritis, gallstones, and nervous conditions. Physician-supervised regimens of milk and rest were thought to help ailing women remain calm, gain strength, and restore fertility. These cures also helped to keep doctors (whose ranks were on the rise) in business. Doctors promulgated the belief that the copious consumption of milk, combined with abundant rest, helped the body to make better blood. Female patients were easily convinced to follow the treatment since milk was viewed as a healthy, healing food, rich in nourishing butterfat. Wealthy women like Kate were supplied with the fresh, highly caloric milk produced by Jersey cows—they were instructed to drink between five and ten quarts of milk daily and rest, take hot baths, and use enemas to avoid constipation.

While Kate convalesced in the south, her health further deteriorated when she developed bronchitis and dysentery. Upon returning home she received a further blow—her grandfather was seriously ill; he passed away soon thereafter in May 1887, leaving Kate and her siblings their father's interest in his estate. Kate described him as "a wonderful grandfather, and although such a busy and sought after man, he always had time to hear anything of interest to us children."[4]

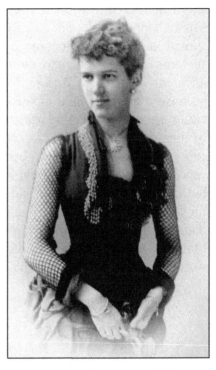

Kate, age 26 *(Courtesy of the Macy Family)*

Notwithstanding the loss of one of her closest family members and intermittent periods of ill health, Kate remembered the seven years that she and Walter passed on Central Park South as a busy and happy time. She filled her days with intellectually stimulating activities as well as involvement with family and friends. Her friend Anna Paret, said that she was "fully devoted to self-culture and mental improvement"[5] and Kate's weekly schedule bears this out.

On Monday mornings she attended Bible class led by the Presbyterian theologian Dr. Charles A. Briggs, an expert in Hebrew and Biblical theology known for controversial beliefs that would lead to his excommunication from the Presbyterian Church. Kate admitted to feeling challenged by his lectures which she considered to be interesting, but "very deep" and at times beyond her realm of understanding.[6] In contrast to the difficulties she associated with Dr. Briggs, Kate found her other classes to be heartening. Her Wednesday morning Current Events classes with Miss Brown were "most delightful" and perhaps it was through her attendance at Mr. Stoddard's travel lectures where he "threw" pictures on a screen that she was inspired to travel abroad again.[7]

Kate's Friday evenings were particularly sociable as she and her
sister were devoted to learning to play the popular game of Whist. Her
teacher was Miss Gertrude Clapp, "one of the earliest and foremost
lady teachers of the game."[8] As such, her talent was in great demand.
Miss Clapp was in an enviable position as a single woman. She
earned. a significant income by teaching fifteen classes each week;
she enjoyed her work and said that it was "an excitement to find the
different avenues to different minds, a problem which never tires,
because it is so difficult to solve."[9] Miss Clapp's classes were held at
either Kate or Mae's apartment. One can picture a group of eight
women gathering for their lesson on West Fifty-Eighth Street, perhaps
enjoying a light supper of Lobster Newburgh and celery salad, wafers,
cheese, and coffee before beginning their lesson in earnest. After Kate
bid farewell to her teacher and fellow students she eagerly turned in
for the night; within a few hours it was time to rise and prepare for her
Saturday morning Shakespeare class conducted by Miss Hallock at
Mae's apartment. Kate admired her teacher and said that the classes
were so outstanding that she never skipped a single one.

Chapter 15

Throughout her tenure on West Fifty-Eighth Street, Kate maintained a busy pace dividing her time between New York City and her mother's estate at Irvington. On occasion she and Walter traveled to visit faraway family such as her cousin Cornelia (Bunnie) Macy Harris, her husband, and baby at their home in Kansas City. While she was thrilled by the visit, Kate continued to struggle as more and more of the women in her circle embraced motherhood.

Kate suffered the indignity of her childless state silently. Although women might count on each other for support, they were reluctant to talk about their personal problems with men. Their husbands typically shied away from discussing female matters and while the average male doctor felt comfortable attending a woman's physical symptoms, he was less likely to address her emotional needs. In Kate's day, medical men matter-of-factly stressed that "miscarriage" or "spontaneous abortion" was such a common occurrence that it was a natural part of reproduction, small comfort to a woman who was unable to carry a child to term.

One wonders whether Kate ever considered consulting a woman doctor who may have offered her greater compassion. In all likelihood she did not; affluent men often held the view that even those women doctors on staff at prestigious hospitals were best suited to run immigrant dispensaries and focus on the treatment of poor women and children. Simply put, men viewed women who practiced medicine to be inferior to their male counterparts. Since Walter managed all matters related to Kate's health, the decision regarding whom to consult was in his hands. Nevertheless, without her husband's knowledge, she probably sampled some of the popular and readily available health tonics of the day such as Mrs. Lydia Estes Pinkham's Vegetable Compound, a patent medicine purported to promote fertility and assuage nervousness. Pinkham's product was a concoction of herbs, roots, and alcohol; the label on the bottle proclaimed that the elixir contained fifteen percent alcohol "added solely as a solvent and preservative." Lydia Pinkham became a wealthy woman as a result of the desperation of women such as Kate.

Kate began to suffer from insomnia in 1890 as she continued to grapple with her inability to conceive. By this time, Mae was distracted by her duties as the mother of two small boys. As Kate agonized over the fact that she might never provide Walter with an heir, she found a caring and devoted friend in her new sister-in-law, Rebecca Humphrey Serrill. Rebecca, who was called "Rebe," married Walter's brother, Jim, on October 9, 1889; the couple had been introduced by Rebe's brother Will who, like Jim, was an engineer.

Rebe was a godsend to Kate. The summer after Rebe married Jim, she and Kate enjoyed a two-week holiday with their husbands in the woods of Poland, Maine. While the men fished and hiked, the women had the opportunity to become well-acquainted. The women were both intelligent and found that they could discuss a wide range of subjects as well as share their deepest feelings.

Since they were both raised in the homes of ardent Friends, Quaker values informed much of their thinking. Nevertheless, the sisters-in-law represented different worlds. Kate was a city mouse whose life had always revolved around society and the excitement of New York, while Rebe was a country mouse from Darby, Pennsylvania, a quiet and close-knit community dominated by the Quaker meetinghouse, school, and burial ground. Kate's family brownstone was one of many such dwellings on an impersonal stretch of Fifty-Third Street; passersby could be from almost anywhere. In contrast, the Serrill home faced Main Street, and from the vantage point of her front garden gate Rebe could easily observe the comings and goings of relatives, friends, and neighbors, people who helped to shape her kind and trusting nature.

Despite having grown up in such diametrically opposed physical environments, the women had much in common, foremost being their love of learning. Kate valued education, and as we have learned she took a variety of classes that stimulated her mind. Her sister-in-law also understood the need for mental stimulation; she was a voracious reader and constant diarist. Kate realized that Rebe was as well-read as Julia Nott and Miss Hallock when she showed Kate a small red book entitled *What Shall I Read?* Here Rebe maintained a meticulous record of every book she had read from age fifteen, entering each book's title, author, date completed, and a remark. Her first entry was "The (sic) Tale of Two Cities" by Charles Dickens about which she commented, "Strongly written, London and Paris are the two cities." As book lovers, the women always had something interesting to discuss. When on holiday they explored new literary horizons together, finding comfort in reading aloud; they loved the sound of each other's voices. Even amidst the hustle and bustle of the train station they perched on unforgiving benches with luggage piled at their feet, content to tackle *The Newcomes* by William Makepeace Thackeray ("Very fine") and Victor Hugo's *Notre Dame* ("Very exciting but unsatisfactory ending") while their impatient husbands paced up and down the platform and consulted their pocket watches.

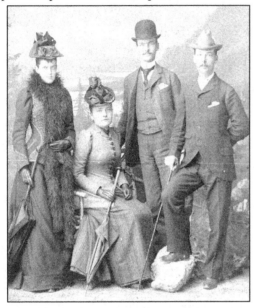

Visiting the Swiss Alps in 1891: Kate, Rebecca Serrill and James B. Ladd, and Walter Ladd *(Courtesy of Frances Ladd Hundt)*

Jim Ladd decided to take his wife abroad in January 1891. He told his brother Walter that he was going to Europe for his health. The exact nature of his poor health is not known; however, since Jim was able to maintain a busy travel schedule in Europe it is plausible that his infirmity was a result of work-related strain sometimes called "tired nerves."

Since Walter had retired from business and was living the leisurely life of a gentleman, the Ladds decided to join Jim and Rebe on the continent. The couples rendezvoused in London in May and they spent what Kate recalled as "five delightful months in Europe; a never to be forgotten trip."[1] Aware of their preference for first-rate accommodations, Jim and Rebe secured rooms for Kate and Walter at

the Hotel Savoy, situated between the Strand and the Thames and
known to be frequented by stage stars and members of the aristocracy.
The Savoy, which had opened in 1889, was the talk of the town, and
everyone who was anyone was agog over the hotel's unique
amenities, which included full electrification, hot water night and day,
and matchless cuisine. The dining room's bill of fare was touted to be
the best in town due to the painstaking management of Mr. Cesar Ritz
and his talented head-chef Monsieur Auguste Escoffier. However,
since Jim was in the habit of counting his pennies, he and Rebe
lodged in a less opulent hotel nearby. Nevertheless, they dined as a
foursome, sometimes on the Savoy's open-air terrace where they

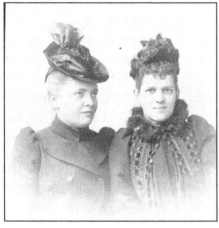

could view the Embankment
Gardens and watch a constant
parade of vessels gliding by on
the Thames.

The Ladd men and their
wives made a compatible group.
When the brothers peeled off to
sightsee, the women happily
entertained themselves, reading,
sewing, shopping, and having
what they called "their little
talks." Kate recognized that some
of Rebe's clothing was in need of
replacement and encouraged her
to visit a dressmaker. Always
practical Rebe went so far as to
order a mackintosh and a sturdy

Rebecca (Rebe) and Kate in their
fashionable hats *(Courtesy of
Frances Ladd Hundt)*

cloth overcoat. Kate who loved fashion (and considered her sister-in-
law's attire dowdy for such a young woman) insisted that, at the very
least, she select a special hat. With Kate's help, Rebe chose
something stylish and gay at Ritchies in London.

Wearing their fashionable chapeaus, Kate and Rebe accompanied
their husbands to the Isle of Wight where they passed ten pleasant
days. The party stayed at the Royal Marine Hotel; they had reserved
adjoining rooms and shared a cozy little sitting room. Rebe noted in
her diary that it was so nice to be together, and Kate happily
remembered their beautiful excursions in a four-in-hand coach. After

lunch on May 27, the women donned their hats and made their way to
Maison Rouge, 31 High Street in Ventnor. This was the home and
studio of local photographer Samuel J. Porter who had been in
business for a few years. His studio was highly successful,
notwithstanding a fair amount of competition, and it remained in the
family when his sister Sarah took charge after his death in 1913.

Porter's charming photograph renders an image of two
dramatically different-looking women. Kate is angular, dark-haired
and slender; her attire is elaborate—ribbons and fur and pearl ear bobs
complemented by fashionably coiffed hair and a Parisian hat. Rebe,
on the other hand, looks soft and round; she is blonde and her downy
hair is swept back simply and tucked up beneath her pretty new hat.
Her coat is well made—serviceable and lacking in adornment. The
women look as different as night and day, every bit city mouse and
country mouse. Even though no one would ever mistake them for
sisters, in their hearts Kate and Rebe keenly felt the loving bond of
sisterhood.

While Jim and Walter seemed to be invigorated by constant
travel, Rebe and Kate were often tired. When they returned to London
they consulted with Dr. Playfair, a well-known women's physician
and colleague of Dr. T. Gaillard Thomas. Kate's chief symptom was
dizziness. Upon careful examination Dr. Playfair said, "You are very
much rundown and in my opinion will never be well until you have
the 'rest cure.'" Kate unequivocally told him, "I have not come
abroad to go to bed. I have a busy schedule of travel planned for
myself."[2] But in this era it was conventionally accepted that humans
possessed a finite amount of energy and that women in particular
were prone to energy depletion. Therefore, Kate and Rebe agreed to
rest in between activities. When Rebe required rest they relaxed
together and Kate read aloud or they talked or sewed. When Kate felt
used up they followed the same routine, and Rebe did the reading. Jim
and Walter seemed to take pride in their wives' delicacy, and they
bantered back and forth about which woman was the greater invalid,
as if being the protective husband of a weak female made one more of
a man.

In Paris the women continued to intersperse rest with touring.
Some mornings they were content to answer letters from home,
crochet, and chat while the men set off walking, Jim with his camera

in hand. He was an amateur photographer and in the evenings he would often disappear for hours to develop his plates. While he was gone, Walter conversed with other men and Rebe and Kate played Whist. Sometimes they visited with folks from home such as the men's uncle Samuel Ladd, who lived in London off and on, and Theodora Van Wyck from Brooklyn. As we recall it was "Dora" who changed the trajectory of Kate's life when she introduced her to Walter at Richfield Springs. Kate lamented that her friend was heading for spinsterhood—her widowed mother relied on her for companionship and discouraged her from meeting eligible men. Kate feared that Dora might wither away in the company of Mrs. Van Wyck and her circle of elderly friends.

Though the details remained a mystery, the issue of Jim's health arose suddenly as the couples progressed through Europe. He was feeling poorly, and a doctor instructed him to seek a higher altitude for his health. Conversely, Kate was told to avoid the mountains on account of her dizzy spells. As a result, when Jim and Rebe went to St. Moritz, high in the snow-capped Alps, Kate and Walter headed to Ragatz, the Swiss spa town, which Kate recognized from the pages of Johanna Spyri's charming novel *Heidi*. Kate indulged in calming baths; the thermal waters were crystal clear and odor free, a pleasant change from the pungent sulfur springs she had previously encountered at health resorts. Even so, she found the daily bath regimen tiresome, and it was not until she had completed a four-week course of treatment that she was told that it was safe for her to join Rebe and Jim at St. Moritz. One might speculate that the four weeks at Ragatz were of greater financial benefit to the doctor who oversaw the resort than of medical benefit to Kate.

Rebe was thrilled to be reunited with Kate, and she greeted her with a large bouquet of field flowers that she and Jim had picked together. The women had a lot to catch up on but they did not dwell either on Kate's or Jim's health. Rebe was far more concerned about the well-being of her sister Frances, who had contracted typhoid fever, the disease that was responsible for Kate's father's death. Rebe knew that her sister was receiving good care at home in Darby and Kate did her best to put Rebe at ease. The younger woman focused much of her energy on her crocheting; she was making a warm woolen shawl to send to her sister.

During those days at St. Moritz the women kept busy but in a leisurely way. They walked in the woods, picked bunches of wildflowers, watched tennis matches at their hotel, listened to music and talked. Rebe read *Childhood, Boyhood and Youth* by Tolstoy aloud to Kate, and come evening they played Whist, read, or wrote letters. Upon their return to Paris, the Ladd brothers began to make travel arrangements. Jim quickly arranged passage home since Rebecca was increasingly concerned about her ailing sister; he knew that she would remain uneasy until she and Frances were reunited. On the other hand, Walter and Kate were not in a rush to go home and so they lingered in France for several more weeks. By the time they docked in New York in November 1891, they had received word that Rebecca's sister Frances Serrill was on the mend. Kate was heartened by the good news; however, her sense of relief was fleeting because she was soon to learn that her own dear sister's health was in great jeopardy.

Chapter 16

MAE MACY WILLETS DISCOVERED A LUMP IN HER BREAST early in 1892, shortly before the birth of her third son, Valentine. Initially the protuberance was the size of a large pearl, but she did not feel distressed. Instead she rubbed the area with salve and engaged a wet nurse for her infant. Nevertheless, the tumor continued to grow. By early May, it had grown so large that Kate was alarmed and persuaded her to see Dr. Thomas. After a thorough examination he concluded that Mae's condition was exceedingly serious and that she required an operation without delay. Kate immediately engaged two rooms at the doctor's sanitarium at 596 Lexington Avenue so that she could remain by Mae's side, knowing that her sister faced a cruel and grueling ordeal.

The Macys were panic-stricken; no one knew much about breast removal surgery except that it was barbaric, disfiguring, and agonizingly painful, and that ultimately a high percentage of women did not survive the procedure. To everyone's dismay the operation proved to be even more involved than anticipated, and in three weeks' time additional surgery was necessary to remove lumps from under Mae's arm. All told, she and Kate spent five weeks together in the sanitarium. Kate commented that as hard as this experience was she considered it to be a great privilege to stay by her sister's side. Mae remarked that she did not know what she would have done without Kate's steadfast presence.

Kate never forgot the kindness that Dr. Thomas and others extended to her and her sister throughout their stay at "596." During the first few days and nights post-surgery, Thomas was not certain that Mae would survive. However, he assured Kate that he would be in constant touch and told her that he kept a telephone beside his bed so that he could be reached at a moment's notice. Kate's physician, Dr. Porter Flewellyn Chambers, came in to visit regularly and did much to keep her courage up, but he never tried to deceive her about the seriousness of her sister's condition. Dr. Sam Lambert, the husband of Howard's sister Bessie, was an up and coming physician; he visited his sister-in-law daily. Mae had tremendous confidence in him and correctly predicted that he would make a great name for himself one day. As the weeks progressed, Kate's health was also affected, and an attending physician told her that her pulse was

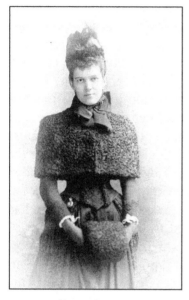

weaker than her sister's. He warned Kate that she could not continue to care for her sister without jeopardizing her own health, an admonition that would come to pass.

At the end of June Kate and Mae left the sanitarium and went to stay at Carrie's country house. Mae would linger at Greystone for almost a year, unable to leave the property and in constant physical and emotional pain.

In July, Kate's family physician insisted that if she stayed with her sister any longer she would completely break down and become an added care to their mother. He told her that if she went to Schwalbach, Germany and took a cure she might get well and would consequently be of greater help to her

Kate, age 29 *(Courtesy of the Macy Family)*

family. With each passing day Kate understood that her sister's condition was hopeless, yet she was reluctant to leave. It was Mae who persuaded her to go abroad. Kate left her sister with the heaviest of hearts and said that she could not have felt worse had Mae been her own baby, so dependent had the older sister become on the younger. Kate's farewell was to be her final goodbye to Mae, for she "never saw her again in this world."[1] When the Ladds returned from Europe Mae was no longer fully conscious.

Kate and Walter sailed on the *Aller* and went directly to Schwalbach where they were met by the Kingslands. The town of Schwalbach, like Richfield and Saratoga Springs, was known for iron infused water. Scrawny women strolled about the various health spas sipping water from small china cups or took advantage of the mineral

baths—what the doctors called "balneological" procedures. Kate was
under the care of Dr. Bohem, whom she called a kind-hearted and
clever physician. He found her to be anemic, and he understood that
she suffered from badly frayed nerves due to her recent experience as
her sister's caregiver and witness to her irreversible decline. When
Kate collapsed after a few treatments and remained in a state of
paralysis for three days Dr. Bohem did not panic. He viewed Kate to
be a neurasthenic like many of the highly strung upper-class women
who frequented the spa. Kate cooperated with Bohem's repetitive
treatment; she knew that her nerves were shattered and required
complete repair so that she could be helpful to her mother. She had let
Carrie down by marrying against her wishes and having difficulties
after her miscarriage. Kate did not want to fail her mother again.

Kate improved gradually, and when her hotel was about to close
for the season she decided to move on to England before facing the
Atlantic crossing. The Ladds went to Tunbridge Wells near London
where Kate could continue to rebuild her stamina as well as visit her
former "596" companion Nettie Warner whose husband William had
recently passed away in France. Out of sight from the New York press
and local gossips, Nettie was beginning to rebuild her life. As a
widow she had become quite dependent upon her secretary, Mr.
James Masters, a former clergyman who was now a boarder at the
Warner home. Several years later, Kate was not at all surprised to
learn that Nettie and Mr. Masters had married.

James Masters helped the Ladds secure passage home on the
steamship *Majestic*. Howard Willets met them at the New York
pier—his face was pinched, and he was as thin as a rail, which told
Kate that her sister's condition was desperate. The realization that
Mae was not long for the world was more than Kate could handle; she
fainted on the ship's gangplank and had to be carried off. Kate
remained in bed for days at the Hotel Loggiot on lower Fifth Avenue.
Tan bark was laid on the street to quiet the noise of horse hooves on
the cobblestone so that she could rest more peacefully.

When Kate returned to her apartment she learned that Mae
moved in and out of consciousness and no longer asked for her
children. Kate joined her closest family members and Mary
Kingsland's minister to stand vigil in Mae's darkened room; she
could not tear herself from her sister's side even though her suffering,

temporarily relieved by liberal doses of the morphine, was unbearable to witness. Mae was suspended in another world. One can imagine Kate's offer of small mercies as she tried her best to comfort her dying loved one: reading cherished poems from childhood days, mopping her brow with a cool lilac scented handkerchief, softly stroking her lifeless hand.

By January Carrie and Everit were on the verge of collapse. Kate was determined to be brave and minister to Mae. To this end she spent day after day by her bedside, suffused with worry, barely eating or sleeping. Consequently, she suffered a calamitous breakdown as her Aunt Mary would note in her diary,

> Tis a sad winter. My darling niece is a sufferer in the widest sense of the word since her terrible operation last May. All these months she has been living a life of daily agony, which causes our hearts to ache almost breaking. Dear child how she tried to be patient and rest in the love of God. When she asks my prayers for this to end, fearing she may not be as patient as she might be I realize how indeed it is only God who can sustain her in these trying hours. We do indeed add our prayers to hers for His tender mercy and loving help.
>
> Kate is now in Philadelphia trying to regain her health, which is sadly shattered.
>
> Mary Jane Macy Kingsland

Dr. Chambers recommended that she see Dr. Silas Weir Mitchell, the preeminent Philadelphia physician who specialized in nervous disorders. He was best known for his "Rest Cure," and he developed the regimen to cure women of an illness called neurasthenia. Wealthy women like Kate who were prone to breaking down under strain were his prime patients.

By the 1870s American physicians had successfully created a diagnostic profile for nervous exhaustion—Dr. Edwin H. Van Deusen and Dr. George M. Beard are credited independently with coining the term neurasthenia for what might otherwise have been referred to as nervous prostration or a case of nerves. In 1869 Beard officially introduced "neurasthenia" to his peers in an article titled "Neurasthenia, or Nervous Exhaustion" published in the *Boston Medical and Surgical Journal*. He publicly presented his findings to the New York Medical Journal Association.[2]

Beard said,

In this country, nervous exhaustion (neurasthenia) is more common than any other kind of nervous disease. With the various neuroses to which it is allied, and to which it leads, it constitutes a family of functional disorders that are of comparatively recent development, that abound in the northern and eastern part of the United States. The term, itself, derives from the Greek and literally means lack of nerve strength.[3]

By the early 1890s neurasthenia had become a catch-all diagnosis that covered a raft of symptoms including fatigue, poor appetite, weight loss, muscle and joint pain, irritability, impotence, insomnia and general anxiety: Neurasthenia was referred to as a "household word" by the dawn of the twentieth century because the diagnosis had become so pervasive. Doctors told patients that their poor health was due to a case of nervous exhaustion, an unpleasant consequence of the hectic pace of urban life. Neurasthenia was said to particularly afflict individuals whose lives were stretched thin by responsibilities associated with work, community, and family.[4]

"Neurasthenics" believed that their symptoms were caused by a physical disorder, exhausted nerves, not by a mental or emotional weakness. To shore up their contentions Beard and his colleagues offered a theory of mental and physical health derived from archaic assumptions about bodily energy, suggesting that humans were infused with a specific amount of "nerve force" or nervous energy. When the body's supply of nerve force was taxed too heavily by the demands of modern life and not adequately replenished a nervous bankruptcy resulted. Doctors based their assertion that neurasthenia generally struck men and women with refined sensibilities on the prevailing nineteenth century concept of Social Darwinism, contending that the elite possessed more highly evolved nervous systems than members of the lower classes. Much of what doctors agreed upon and told their patients about illness in Kate's day strikes us today as far-fetched and implausible; contemporary medical historians are quick to point out that what represented science prior to the twentieth century was not necessarily clear or accurate.[5]

Class and gender fully dictated a neurasthenic's course of treatment. Male sufferers were instructed to follow the "West Cure" and enjoy life in the great outdoors—hunting, fishing, riding, climbing mountains, and bonding with other men in order to build themselves back up for continued success in business and intellectual pursuits.[6] Women, on the other hand, were instructed to seek the "Rest Cure" through confinement and isolation. It is worth noting that nerve specialists catered to the well-off who were their bread and butter. When poor women complained of fatigue, anxiety, body pain, insomnia, or other symptoms that comprised the catch-all of neurasthenia, they were labeled hysterics. If their complaints were too loud or their behavior too unruly they chanced being committed to the asylum.[7]

Silas Weir Mitchell, recognized as the father of American neurology, developed a keen interest in neurasthenia. Between 1870 and 1914 he maintained a lucrative medical practice in Philadelphia. Over the years, many words and phrases have been uttered to describe him: He was called a brilliant physician, a successful novelist, a pillar of the community as well as a short-tempered, greedy, and misogynistic person. To Kate, however, he became a rare and treasured friend.

Mitchell was a man of high achievement in his era. Born in 1829, he was a native Philadelphian and third generation medical doctor who had enrolled at the University of Pennsylvania at the age of fifteen and earned a medical degree from Thomas Jefferson Medical College several years later. Thereafter, he studied in Europe, working with the French physician and "father" of physiology, Claude Bernard. He returned to Philadelphia to practice medicine with his father, simultaneously embarking upon a career in scientific research; this resulted in the publication of more than one hundred books and articles; twenty-five papers appeared in the *Proceedings of the American Academy of Natural Sciences of Philadelphia* between 1853 and 1870 alone. It was during this period that Mitchell became interested in the field of neurology in large part due to his experience treating wounded veterans.[8]

Mitchell always practiced in Philadelphia; he spent the years of the Civil War (during which some 620,000 soldiers died) working as a contract surgeon at Turner's Lane Hospital, a 400-bed army hospital that specialized in nervous diseases. In an attempt to save lives, Union and Confederate surgeons including Mitchell had performed more than 50,000 amputations, which left countless men permanently disabled.[9] Through his work, Mitchell encountered scores of veterans who had suffered traumatic nerve injuries. This provided him with an unprecedented opportunity to study nerve-related disorders on a large scale and led to the publication of *Gunshot Wounds and Other Injuries of Nerves* which he co-authored with two fellow army surgeons. This groundbreaking work remained the most authoritative source on nerve injuries in the world for more than one hundred years.[10]

By the conclusion of the war Mitchell had become a respected authority on nervous diseases; he returned to a civilian practice to focus on this medical specialty. In 1870, he was appointed "Physician" to the two-room Philadelphia Orthopedic Hospital for Nervous Diseases where he remained on staff for more than forty years—under his leadership the hospital grew into one of the foremost centers for the treatment of nervous disease in the United States with public hospital wards and three dozen private rooms.

In 1871, Mitchell's focus shifted somewhat. He published a revised edition of his work on gunshot wounds and turned his attention toward the treatment of nervous illnesses as recently defined by George Beard. Within two years he published a book intended for the general public, *Wear and Tear or Hints for the Overworked.* It was so well-received that the first edition sold out in ten days. The volume addressed such topics as diet, exercise, and the need for rest, elements that had been part of Mitchell's course of treatment for veterans. Mitchell's book resonated with his readers and brought him a plethora of inquiries from nervous women who sought medical treatment. This led him to understand that a medical treatment for neurasthenia was suddenly the "taste of the hour."[11]

Mitchell's realization of the opportunity that lay within his reach led to the publication of his most seminal work, *Fat and Blood,* in 1877—a book-length essay about the management of neurasthenia. This work came to overshadow his more scientifically based research in the field of neurology and forever identified him with the rest cure. In *Fat and Blood* he explained that nervous patients, typically well-off women who were thin and excitable, needed to add body weight and renew red blood cells by consuming foods high in fat in order to restore health. He logically posited that this result could best be achieved by keeping a patient at rest—in bed and unable to exert energy and burn calories. Mitchell's cure was comprised of five critical elements: rest, seclusion, food, massage, and electricity; the regimen would best be managed by a trained nurse. Here we have the foundation of the Mitchell Rest Cure, which Dr. Chambers thought would be beneficial to Kate in the winter of 1893.

Fat and Blood

For some years, I have been using with success, in private and in hospital practice, certain methods of renewing the vitality of feeble people by a combination of entire rest and excessive feeding, made possible by passive exercise obtained through the steady use of massage and electricity.

The cases thus treated have been chiefly women of a class well known to every physician, nervous women, who, as a rule, are thin and lack blood. Most of them have been such as had passed through many hands and been treated in turn for gastric, spinal, or uterine troubles, but who remained at the end as at the beginning, invalids, unable to attend to the duties of life, and sources alike of discomfort to themselves and anxiety to others.

A woman, most often between twenty and thirty years of age, undergoes a season of trial or encounters some prolonged strain. She may have undertaken the hard task of nursing a relative, and have gone through this severe duty with the addition of emotional excitement swayed by hopes and fears and forgetful of self and of what everyone needs in the way of air and food and change when attempting this most trying task. In another set of cases an illness is the cause and she never rallies entirely, or else some local uterine trouble starts the mischief, and although this is cured, the doctor wonders that his patient does not get fat and ruddy again.[12]

One of the questions of most importance in the carrying out of this treatment (the rest cure) is the choice of nurse…The nurse for these cases ought to be a young, active, quick-witted woman, capable of firmly but gently controlling her patient. She ought to be intelligent, able to interest her patient, to read aloud, and to write letters.[13]

Walter met with Dr. Mitchell at his office at 524 Walnut Street in Philadelphia. When he returned to New York a few days later, he was accompanied by one of Mitchell's best young nurses, Miss Alice Lemley.

Kate remarked that from the moment Miss Lemley entered her room, she felt as if an angel had come to nurse her. For the next twenty-five years the women were constant and beloved companions. Kate recalled, "She was only twenty-two years-old when she came to me and her coming into my life just at this time I counted as one of my greatest blessings."[14]

Alice and Kate spent a few days getting acquainted, and then Dr. Chambers and Walter took the women to Philadelphia where they stayed at the Stratford Hotel on Broad Street in order to be under Dr. Mitchell's care. Kate was so thin and weak that Dr. Chambers carried her in his arms whenever she needed to be lifted or moved; he convinced her that the rest cure was her best chance for a full recovery from her shattered nerves.

Chapter 17

KATE'S FIRST ENCOUNTER WITH SILAS WEIR MITCHELL was an eventful and unsettling occasion. They chatted and he examined her thoroughly. When Miss Lemley asked Kate how she liked Dr. Mitchell, she cried and said that she thought he was "horrid" and she continued to think poorly of him for the next five weeks.[1] Kate was desperate to be at Greystone with her sister. She wanted Walter to take her home, but before he agreed to do so he spoke to John Mitchell, who practiced medicine with his father. After their conversation, the younger man intervened. Subsequently, the senior Dr. Mitchell entered Kate's room a changed man. He walked quietly to the side of her bed, from which she had barely been permitted to move for more than a month, gently took her hand and apologized for his behavior saying, "My dear child, I hear I have hurt your feelings, and I would not have done it for anything in the world," to which Kate replied, "Yes, Dr. Mitchell, I felt you thought I was a crank."[2] He indicated that had he thought poorly of her, she would have been told immediately. Thereafter, things improved between doctor and patient and in time they developed a close and enduring friendship.

Despite some of the less pleasant aspects of the rest cure, Dr. Mitchell's patients were spared procedures that typified gynecological treatment in the late nineteenth century. He did not use sedatives or potentially addictive painkillers indiscriminately, nor did he advocate removal of female organs unless completely warranted. Nonetheless, his treatment was physically restrictive—Kate spent her first five weeks of treatment flat on her back with only one small pillow beneath her head. To a woman accustomed to luxury her surroundings were Spartan, and all she was permitted to do for herself was to clean her teeth. She could neither send nor receive letters; therefore, she was in the dark regarding Mae's condition. This was difficult for Kate to accept, but Miss Lemley explained that seclusion was an absolutely necessary element of the cure.

Kate was kept in bed for a full three months; she does not mention whether Walter was permitted to visit her as he had done when she was a patient at the Lexington Sanitarium. We do not know whether she spent her time in a hotel or if she was being cared for in one of the private rooms at the newly enlarged Orthopedic Hospital for Nervous Diseases.

The goal of Mitchell's rest cure was to help women gain fat and blood. Like most of the women under Dr. Mitchell's care, Kate was painfully thin, pale, and anemic. Mitchell postulated that an increase in weight and red blood cells would lead to an improvement in physical and mental health. Therefore, a regimen of complete bed rest was supplemented by a food-heavy diet. As the doctor wrote in *Fat and Blood,* "a gain in fat up to a certain point seems to go hand in hand with a rise in all other essentials of health."[3] Initially, Kate followed a version of the milk diet. She was treated like a baby and spoon-fed large quantities of milk and cream which were expected to add energy and fat to her starved body. After about ten days, she advanced to eating three sizable meals each day, generally starting off with a few ounces of malt extract to stimulate her appetite. This was followed by pints of milk, bread spread with liberal amounts of butter, a mutton chop or oysters, and a dense soup made from one pound of raw chopped beef. Mitchell typically prescribed iron supplements and small doses of strychnine, a known stimulant, which was promoted as an energy tonic as well as arsenic, which enhanced weight gain and stimulated circulation to add rosiness to a sickly woman's ghostly pallor. It is likely that Kate swallowed foul tasting cod liver oil to forestall the added complication of constipation.

As a rest cure patient Kate was expected to be submissive at all times. She was attended by Miss Lemley and two other nurses who helped to bathe and feed her, take her to the toilet, and move her from one position to another to avoid bed sores. Other individuals aided in her care and helped to define the monotonous rhythm of her day. Mrs. Durham, a strong woman well-trained in her art, provided daily massages to stimulate Kate's circulation. Dressed in a crisp white uniform, the masseuse rolled and kneaded the young woman's feet and massaged her entire body. Special care was given to Kate's spine and loins, and over time the massages became more intense. Isolated as she was, Kate may have welcomed the woman's touch. In the absence of physical therapy as practiced today, Dr. Charles Burr quietly appeared each evening to give Kate electrical treatments. The electricity was conducted from a small wooden cabinet, a simple premise as explained by Dr. Burr: A low voltage wire was applied to Kate's leg muscles to make them contract and prevent them from going slack while she was confined to bed. On occasion if a patient was severely constipated electrical stimulation might be ordered— electrodes were placed in the patient's rectum and on the stomach. One would assume that Kate did everything possible to avoid such an agonizing and humiliating circumstance.

Unlike rest cure patient and author Charlotte Perkins Gilman whose 1892 novella, *The Yellow Wallpaper,* portrayed S. Weir Mitchell as a medical misogynist, Kate felt that she benefitted greatly under Mitchell's strictly supervised care. She said that her rest cure was a trying but most necessary experience and claimed that Dr. Mitchell helped her to a "broader, more wholesome view of life" and "new avenues of thought."[4] S. Weir Mitchell was known to radiate charisma. Kate probably viewed him as a father figure; he was tall and strikingly handsome and personable as her own father had been. She was devastated when he passed away in 1914 and claimed that she had lost a perfect friend.

Chapter 18

AN 1893 ISSUE OF SAMUEL MCCLURE'S self-titled literary and political magazine featured an interview with Silas Weir Mitchell, (incorrectly referring to him as Samuel Weir Mitchell) called "Nervousness: The National Disease of America."[1] It explained that neurasthenia was so prevalent among upper-class women that it had spawned a fashionable cult of female invalidism wholly supported by their husbands. The thinking was that if a woman was weak, delicate, and fluttered passively beneath her spouse's patriarchal wing, his reputation would be burnished—he would be praised as protective, devoted, and manly—his needy wife was like a badge of honor. If support of a frail woman made him more the man, this might to some extent help to explain the dynamic that existed between Kate and Walter.

In the heyday of neurasthenia women were eager to discuss their fashionable disease with friends. Men did not hide their wives' condition since a diagnosis of neurasthenia implied refinement and suggested that an expensive doctor had been engaged. Perhaps this is why Walter and Jim chatted about which of their wives was a greater invalid. Fashionable women flocked to consult with specialists like Dr. Mitchell, who conducted one of the world's largest consulting practices focusing specifically on women's nervous disorders, and reportedly earned between $70,000 and $100,000 during his peak years of practice, about two million dollars annually in today's money.

Not all physicians were seduced by thoughts of the riches to be obtained by treating wealthy women, however. By the close of the nineteenth century female physicians, who comprised between four and five percent of all doctors, were expressing unease over the surging number of nervous women being treated by "specialists." For example, Dr. Mary Putnam Jacobi, known to be a brilliant physician and spokesperson for the women's medical movement wrote that women who constantly considered their nerves and were "urged to consider them by well-intentioned but short-sighted advisors" soon became nothing but a "bundle of nerves."[2]

Kate was often referred to as an invalid, especially during the last twenty-five years of her life. One need not look too far to find such references: Her employees recalled her sitting out in the sunshine bundled in fur in a wheeled chair, New Jersey neighbors promulgated the false notion that she was bedridden from the time she and Walter married, and disgruntled descendants (who did not benefit markedly from her estate) circulated spurious accounts about her physical and mental capacities. A relative spread the specious tale that she had been an invalid since age eighteen. The term "invalid" is on its face confusing, the definition being, in part, a function of history. Throughout the nineteenth century, an invalid was someone, typically but not exclusively female, in a state of weakness or with a predisposition to illness but not necessarily bedridden or removed from society, and invalidism was not a permanent state. To the contrary, by the twentieth century an invalid was characterized as someone who remained at home, bedridden, unable to move about freely or engage with society. How could such an individual bring status to a spouse?

Under the care of Alice and Dr. Mitchell, Kate realized that she did not want to remain an invalid, and she was dedicated to regaining her health. In five months with Alice's constant encouragement she gained thirty pounds, and her muscles were in good condition. The women had grown close during the months of her rest cure, and Alice agreed to return to New York with Kate to be her full-time nurse companion.

Before she left Philadelphia, Kate posed for a photographic portrait—perhaps Dr. Mitchell was in the habit of commissioning before and after photos of his patients. Looking robust and confident, she was aglow with good health, a far cry from the pathetic wreck who could not sit up in bed when she first arrived in Philadelphia.

While Kate grew healthy and strong, her precious sister was disintegrating into a pile of skin and bones. In the early 1890s the majority of women who had a breast removed would succumb to their cancer in less than three years, and Mae was no exception. On May

12, 1893, after lingering for more than a year, Mae Macy Willets died at Greystone. She was thirty-three years old.

Mary Kingsland wrote,

Our dear Mae is at rest. She passed away peacefully May 12th, 1893. Through long suffering she was purified and made worthy, and what a lovely example of patient-waiting she is to us. One by one her trials came in her illness and she quietly accepted and tried so hard to be patient and bear all uncomplainingly.

We will miss her out of our life, for she was indeed lovely and grew so dear and affectionate to us, yet these days we offer a psalm of Thanksgiving that she has won the victory and is at peace.

As the days go on we will yearn for her true tender love more and more for there is none to take her place- dear Mary Kingsland Macy Willets.

Yesterday we laid her in Woodlawn, another young life laid low...earth's course finished and the heavenly life begun. We left her in the sunshine, with singing birds, and spring flowers but left her with heavy hearts lonely and sad.

Kate's devastation over her sister's death was compounded when she belatedly learned that her most intimate childhood friend Sallie Whitcomb Sterling, the mother of two little girls, had died of consumption that winter. As a result of her grave sadness over Mae and Sallie and their motherless sons and daughters, Kate lost much of the ground she had gained in Philadelphia, and she resumed her day-to-day routine with a painfully heavy heart.

Between 1887 and 1892 the gracious atmosphere and leisurely pace at Carrie Macy's country estate, Greystone, had provided a comforting retreat from city life for Kate, her family, and their guests. The estate was the scene of great joy when Mae's second son, Josiah Macy Willets, was born there on August 25, 1889. Nevertheless, by the spring of 1893 the house was too tragic a reminder of Mae's prolonged illness and death. Carrie decided to sell the country estate whose happy magic had evaporated along with the spark of Mae's earthly life. In October prominent New York merchant Louis Stern, president of Stern Brothers Department Store, purchased Greystone for $255,000.[3]

Chapter 19

After Mae died Kate was overwhelmed with concern about the well-being of her young nephews who were under the care of their paternal grandmother Amelia Willets. As it was with most men of that time, Howard was ill-equipped to raise his sons on his own and it was expected that he would remarry soon after the prescribed period of mourning had been observed to provide a new mother for his boys. Kate, who felt stigmatized as a married woman without children, adored her sister's boys and longed to raise Jack, Josiah, and Valentine in Mae's place. Walter refused to consider such a plan.

After Kate and Walter disagreed about her nephews, she remained at odds with her husband for some time. In her cheerless state she increasingly sought Miss Lemley's counsel and company. The young nurse had become Kate's anchor that first desolate summer after Mae's death, her constant companion and the angel whose sunny warmth helped soak up her sadness. Alice understood how Kate felt about Mae because she was especially close to her own older sister Lily Ann. Her patience and care took on greater meaning as the gulf between Walter and Kate continued to widen.

In late June, Miss Lemley accompanied the Ladds to the mountains to visit Carrie and Everit at Paul Smith's Hotel. On this occasion the usual pleasures of a summer among the pines provided little succor. Nonetheless, the family remained in the Adirondacks; no one could bear the thought of returning to Greystone. The Kingslands encouraged a complete change of scenery for Carrie and urged her to travel to Europe as they had done following the death of their son Cornelius. Kate's mother agreed. After the sale of Greystone was finalized, the family boarded the *S.S. Majestic* bound for England. The large traveling party was composed of Alice Lemley, Carrie, her maid, her brother Thomas Everit and his wife, their daughter Helen (a favorite cousin of Kate's), Everit and Chester Aldrich (his friend and fellow architecture student), Walter, Kate, and her personal maid.

This was Alice's first occasion to travel on a grand scale, and it stands to reason that despite her sadness Kate would attempt to make it an unforgettable experience for her. Raised in the small railroad town of Parkesburg, Pennsylvania, and educated nearby in Philadelphia, Alice had never ventured far from home. Regardless of what others may have characterized as her parochialism, Alice was highly regarded by Dr. Mitchell, and Kate recognized her as a bright and curious young woman from their first meeting. She and her sister Lily were among the first graduates of the nurse training program at the Philadelphia General Hospital. The young women were determined to support themselves in a meaningful professional occupation, and in those days, for a woman, this meant preparing as a teacher or a nurse.

The Macys' trip abroad was slated to get underway with stays in London and Paris, one of Kate's favorite cities. However, the Parisian weather was so cold and raw that autumn that the group changed plans, seeking warmth and sunshine in southern Italy. While in Naples they secured passage to Egypt on the *Cuba* with stops at Porte Said, Alexandria, and Cairo. The party spent several weeks in Egypt, and as Kate recalled, no one was prepared for this strange new land. Even though the sights were fascinating, the wretched condition of the people left her and Alice in a state of anguish. The extreme poverty they encountered at every turn gnawed at them, stimulating the women to do something helpful. Since they were both nimble with needle and thread, Kate and Alice agreed to sew clothing for the poor, half-clad Egyptians, purchasing the necessary supplies in Cairo. Packages of cloth and notions were loaded onto their rented steamer, *Mena*, in time to embark upon a six-week cruise along the Nile.

The beauty of the Nile was a welcome elixir to the travelers. Kate would never forget her sister or the way she had suffered; nevertheless, floating on the river calmed her. She commented about the beauty of the Nile and "the superb sunsets with the long after-glow of that marvelous golden shade, only seen in Egypt..."[1] Time aboard the little boat was a welcome relief after days spent in the dust and grime of Cairo. However, the group's reverie was broken whenever the *Mena* anchored along the river bank where Kate and the others encountered threadbare, desolate-looking people. Their gaunt faces and sore eyes were an upsetting sight for the affluent New

Yorkers who ate, drank, and slept well throughout their journey. Kate and Alice coped by making simple cotton shirts, trousers, and lightweight shifts that may have reminded Kate of the comfortable summer nightgowns of her childhood. Sewing was a good way to use up what she called her Macy energy, and a focus on the Quaker tenet of doing good for others provided a helpful distraction from concerns that had followed her across the Atlantic. A memorable highlight of this leg of the journey was a side trip to see the famous temple ruins at Luxor and Phyllis. Young boys, whom Carrie called "a wild looking set of humanity," brought donkeys for the party to ride to the ruins, and even though the heat was intense Kate wrote that no words could describe the grandeur of all that she encountered.[2]

On February 10, 1894, the Macy party left Alexandria; when they reached Marseille, the group split up to pursue divergent routes for the winter. While everyone else returned to the Continent, Alice, Kate, and Walter chose a more adventurous destination sailing to North Africa for an interlude in Algiers. Walter may have clambered about the Kasbah and other antiquities, but Kate and Alice took long walks and enjoyed gathering wildflowers which they pressed and made into a book. By this time the women had been together for more than a year, and it appears that Alice could read Kate's emotions and help guide her toward a brighter path if needed.

The time abroad passed with lightning speed, and Kate did not want to forget a thing that she experienced so she maintained a journal, a practice she had developed as a young person. Reading entries from a diary can open the floodgates to memories, happy and sad alike. In 1894 Kate joyfully recorded the news of the birth of her niece Frances Serrill Ladd, Rebe and Jim's daughter. The baby was Rebe's pride and joy and she spared no superlatives to describe the wonders of her infant daughter. Kate's diary further documented that the spring weather was very fine in Paris where Walter engaged a cheery apartment at the centrally located Hotel du Rhin on Rue de la Paix by Place Vendome. Kate was so busy showing Alice the city's iconic sights that her "Baedeker Guide" might have disintegrated from overuse. Although the women were reluctant to leave Paris, Kate agreed to a four-week respite at Schwalbach to prevent herself from overdoing it as she was inclined. As before, she joined scores of health seekers including several of her Aunt Mary's New York society friends. The interlude at Schwalbach was restorative, and after side-trips to Ouchy, the Italian lakes, and Milan, Alice and the Ladds moved on to Venice.

Soon after they arrived, Walter had an accident. According to Kate, it was not serious; nevertheless, he was confined to bed for an entire month. Since there was little that they could do for him, Kate and Alice spent their time exploring the city together.

For Kate the very nature of time may have seemed to shift; it is easy to imagine that she enjoyed the freedom of being on her own after a decade of matrimony. She and Alice traversed the watery environs by gondola, which brought back pleasant memories of her first visit to Venice. The women enjoyed riding out to the Lido late in the afternoon to watch the glorious sunsets, which enhanced the magical beauty of the city of canals. By this time Alice had become a perfect friend to her, much as her sister-in-law Rebe had been. Unlike Rebe, however, Alice was unfettered by a baby and a spouse and the demands of married life, and this lent an air of greater freedom and spontaneity to their relationship.

Kate liked to say that she and Alice were perfectly suited. Among many other things, they shared a love of all God's creatures, especially dogs, cats, and birds, and they always found time to stop and feed the pigeons in St. Mark's Square. This may have been where they first observed the comical antics of a most charming breed of dog, the Volpino. Perhaps watching fashionable Venetian ladies on parade with their frisky pups, Kate imagined how nice it might be to raise a little dog with Alice.

Once Walter had mended Kate and Alice approached a stay in Florence with enthusiasm; Kate was bent on showing Alice the famous art galleries, especially the Uffizi and she commented that day after day they climbed up four flights of stairs in order not to miss one picture. However, by the time they reached Rome, Kate's energy had begun to flag and Alice was alarmed to notice that she was losing weight. She shared her concern in a letter to Dr. Mitchell; he responded that they should return home at once. Kate was disappointed to interrupt their time in Italy but since she considered Mitchell's word to be law, she acquiesced and made plans to return home early. Before doing so, she insisted on going to Paris to say goodbye to her family. Everit was experiencing a delayed reaction to

Mae's illness and death; he was under the care of an American doctor. Unknown to Kate, her mother was having difficulties of her own—she was unable to lift her arm without pain, so she also sought medical treatment. As she reluctantly bid her family farewell Kate had no idea that her upcoming ocean voyage would be fraught with danger that would warrant newspaper headlines and test the mettle of each and every soul on board.

The ship *Teutonic* set sail from Liverpool on January 30, 1895. Upon embarkation the weather was fair and the captain expected to be in New York in no time at all. The *Teutonic* and her twin the *Majestic* (which had conveyed them over to Europe) were highly praised modern marvels. Often referred to as floating palaces, they were more extravagantly appointed than some of the finest mansions on Fifth Avenue.

The ships were known for being both speedy and lavish. The *Teutonic's* expansive midship saloon was topped with a sparkling crystal dome that invited bright rays of sunshine indoors; its banquet hall was artistically decorated with an elaborate Renaissance theme. Bas relief figures of tritons and nymphs rendered in gold and ivory skylarked across the ceiling and up and down the walls in a room brilliantly electrified. Sumptuous revolving couches and chairs, a luxurious novelty, encouraged first class passengers to linger and socialize.

In spite of her wealth Kate did not court exclusivity. She was conscious of the fact that she and Walter traveled like aristocrats, but she was satisfied with simpler things. She may have regarded the opulence that surrounded them on the *Teutonic* to be excessive. Had she inquired about the *Teutonic's* less privileged passengers, those whom she would never meet under the dazzling dome of the ship's massive saloon, she would have been told not to be concerned for the steerage compartment was a model for all ships to emulate. In 1893 officials for the White Star Line proudly claimed that an agreeable variety of accommodations were offered below deck including separate family rooms and quarters solely for women traveling alone. These were overseen by a matron to insure the safety of the single maiden. Furthermore, steerage passengers could make the crossing assured that ventilation below deck was good, hot and cold water was provided, and the lavatories were discreet.[3]

As Kate began to relax and ease into the homeward journey, her tranquility was destroyed by unanticipated foul weather. Fierce Atlantic gales and a blinding snowstorm seemed to come out of nowhere, pitting an energy infused ocean against the *Teutonic*; hail pelted down coating every rope and surface of the ship. With such danger afoot only the crew was permitted on deck. This was not such a great hardship for first class passengers. Despite the rough seas their needs were met and their meals were prepared without interruption (although many were too seasick to eat). The ship's captain, however, refused even a crust of bread. So alarmed was he by the treacherous turn in the weather that he maintained a steady vigil from a command post on the ship's bridge. His passengers were horrified to learn that Captain Cameron developed frostbite as a result of his exposure to the icy winds.

The unusually difficult nature of the crossing came as a surprise to everyone since the *Teutonic* was one of the crown jewels in the White Star Line; her very name implied strength and fortitude. The ship had been designed by the well-known firm of Harland & Wolff of Belfast and launched early in 1889. It was built entirely of steel, weighed approximately 10,000 tons, and was designed to accommodate about 1,350 travelers. She was widely believed to be immune to the vicissitudes of the sea. Given that February was not a popular season for travel there were some 400 men, women, and children on board, half of whom traveled in steerage.

It would seem that towing a lighter than usual load should have enabled the *Teutonic* to race across the sea. Known to be one of the fastest liners in the world, she was part of an exclusive fleet of "Ocean Greyhounds" distinguished for having crossed the Atlantic in six days or less. The ship claimed a place in maritime history in the summer of 1892 when she achieved the remarkable run of 528 knots in a single day or the equivalent of an astonishing thirty-three miles per hour. Kate's trip, however, was not to be a record breaking crossing; the inclement weather prolonged the voyage by days. Captain Cameron had expected to reach Sandy Hook along the New Jersey coast at midnight on Tuesday, February 5; his estimated time of arrival was revised repeatedly. New batches of storms were encountered as he advanced the ship toward the mainland. A seasoned officer told a bereft assemblage of passengers that he had never encountered such extreme weather in all his years at sea. With the monstrously high seas, gale force winds, churning waters, and intense cold the trip was in a class of its own. Adding insult to injury, as the *Teutonic* gingerly approached the eastern seaboard the temperature had plunged below zero.

News about the liner's delay was widely covered in the press, alerting the public that further danger had beset the ship before she finally docked at the North River Pier, ten days after setting off from Queenstown, Ireland. It was reported that as the ship came within striking distance of Sandy Hook, New Jersey, a snow-laden hurricane materialized. It was of such ferocity that the bright twin beacons of the Navesink Light Station were obscured; the *Teutonic* had no light to guide her home. Having no choice the ship's veteran captain turned her around, heading seventy miles out to open sea to avoid running aground in the blinding storm. During this episode the ship's telegraphic communication was severed and gigantic waves crashed on deck creating a deafening roar, exacerbated by the constant woeful blast of the foghorn. One crew member was seriously injured when a wave threw him into a windlass. Kate may have wondered how her great-grandfather had managed to successfully navigate the ocean for so many decades, commanding vessels that were far less seaworthy than the *Teutonic*.

After the "floating palace" rolled up and down on the open sea for an entire day, Captain Cameron prepared to make another run toward Sandy Hook. As the *Teutonic* approached the shore, however, a member of the crew set his sights on a small boat bobbling in distress. The *Josie Reeves*, a fishing schooner and her crew were sinking fast; the larger vessel came to their aid with a recovery operation that took most of the day.

The *Josie Reeves* had set out from Brooklyn's Fulton Market a few days before the *Teutonic* had quit Liverpool and encountered bad weather from the start. Nonetheless, the crew fished with fair luck for most of the week, returning to shore briefly to place their ailing cook in quarantine before setting out again. On day eleven of their voyage a terrific eastern gale accompanied by blinding snow also overtook them, compelling their captain to anchor near Sandy Hook. By the next morning, the boat had broken loose from its mooring and was drifting. The schooner was sheathed in ice from stem to stern, and the crew believed that the ice and wind would crush their vessel like it was an eggshell. As the boat took on water the fishermen worked desperately to remain afloat. They were frozen, exhausted, and on the verge of giving up when the *Teutonic* arrived. The drama did not end immediately—the big ship's rescue effort was hard-won due to the relentlessly high seas. The fishermen were eventually intercepted and hoisted up onto the *Teutonic's* deck. The bedraggled crew was welcomed with wild cheers and the ship's chaplain's prayer of Thanksgiving, after which the men graciously accepted whiskey, dry clothing, hot food, and warm beds.[4]

Chapter 20

DURING THE UNEXPECTEDLY EVENTFUL ATLANTIC CROSSING, Kate's mind was too occupied to grapple with the issue that had prompted her abrupt return to New York: Dr. Mitchell's concern about her health. However, after a brief stay at the Waldorf Hotel, Alice and the Ladds traveled to Philadelphia where Mitchell sent Kate to see Dr. Charles Bingham Penrose, a noted gynecologist and the chairman of the Department of Gynecology at the University of Pennsylvania. Kate thought he was a very clever man. Penrose advised her to undergo surgery to correct some congenital trouble. Although it was not considered to be a serious operation, Kate suffered what she called "tortures" for five weeks because a surgical assistant inadvertently cut into her flesh causing two slow-healing wounds. Dr. Mitchell supervised her recovery, and in mid-May 1895 she was finally well enough to move on to Morristown, New Jersey, for a month of further convalescence.

To aid in his wife's recuperation and provide pleasant surroundings for himself, Walter had taken a one-year lease on the Albert Vernam house situated on a broad avenue of millionaires' elegant homes at 101 Madison Avenue in Morristown. The Ladds first learned of the town's many charms from their good friends Adelaide McAlpin and James Tolman Pyle. Addie was an old chum from New York City as well as one of Kate's Richfield Springs summer friends. Her husband James was a well-heeled and easygoing fellow who was known to thoroughly enjoy the high life.

Like Kate, "Frances" Adelaide McAlpin Pyle had been raised in an affluent family. Her father, David H. McAlpin was an industrialist who introduced the mild Virginia strain of tobacco to the smoking public and made millions. His vast wealth provided his sons and daughter with two fine residences—a townhouse on Fifth Avenue, right around the corner from Carrie's house as well as a country estate

called Glen Alpin located due west of Morristown. Adelaide McAlpin
Pyle possessed many unique traits for a woman of her station; she was
both formidably intelligent and driven, the lone female raised in a
household dominated by a band of competitive siblings, all of whom
were Princeton and Yale men. A fine linguist and leading proponent
of nursery school education, she was also the mother of six children.
Her husband, James, was engaged in his family's business
manufacturing "Pyle's Pearline," a popular washing detergent. In
those days one could barely pick up a magazine without noticing an
advertisement for the washing compound which was touted as the
"finest" available and "capable of cleaning laundry, oil paintings and
anything in-between."[1] When the Pyles were in residence at their
country house, "Hurstmont" (located next to David McAlpin's New
Jersey estate), James commuted to New York from the Morristown
train station.

The Ladds felt at home in Morristown, a locale that boasted
tremendous panache. Prior to the 1880s, Morristown had been but a
small village, albeit one that was steeped in history. Early settlers
came in search of iron ore and their mining success furnished a
reliable supply of ore. During the Revolutionary War General George
Washington's troops twice wintered outside of town, enduring great
hardship, close by the land that would eventually become the Glen
Alpin estate. In 1838, Alfred Vail, the son of a local industrialist,
along with inventor Samuel B. Morse, developed a telegraph machine
in the vicinity at the Speedwell Iron Works. Once dependable train
service was established between Morristown and New York City,
wealthy New Yorkers started to buy property and build handsome
homes in the area. It was said that more wealthy men resided within a
three-mile radius of the Ladds' rented home than anywhere;
Morristown was "the core of the richest and least known colony of
wealthy people in the world."[2] It was the stock market crash of 1929
that altered Morristown's veneer of extraordinary wealth as many
opulent properties became too costly to maintain. Subsequently, many
of Morristown's finest mansions were either razed or transformed into
more practical entities such as schools, tract housing developments,
apartment complexes, office buildings, and parks. In the early 1950s
when the Morristown Memorial Hospital was relocated from Morris
Street and reincarnated as a modern hospital it was built across the

street from the original site of the Vernam's Madison Avenue house. By the advent of the twenty-first century, only a handful of the original mansions were still standing, fleeting reminders of Morristown's Gilded Age past.

While the Ladds found life in Morristown to be agreeable, as the summer heat mounted they sought respite at Cooper Camp on Upper St. Regis Lake in the Adirondacks, staying there through October. Charmingly rustic, Cooper was one of the best camps in the North Woods; Kate's summer retreat was a far cry from the elegant Vernam house: her camp accommodation was a fully furnished canvas tent set upon a wooden platform. Meals were served in a dining hall that resembled one found at an informal country hotel.

It was while she was in the Adirondacks that Kate likely made the acquaintance of two individuals who would serve as great inspirations in the future: Dr. Edward Livingston Trudeau and Mrs. Elizabeth Milbank Anderson. The doctor cared for consumptives and conducted important medical research at his sanitarium at Saranac Lake and Mrs. Anderson was one of his most ardent supporters. Thousands of people were dying of consumption annually; most of those who succumbed to tuberculosis like Kate's dear friend Sallie Whitcomb Sterling were struck down in the prime of life. Kate was intrigued to learn about Dr. Trudeau's "constant friends," an assembly of well-heeled men and women who pledged financial support to his hospital the "Adirondack Cottage Sanitarium" as well as his research efforts.

Having spent twenty-two months traveling around Europe, Everit and Carrie returned to New York. When they visited Kate in the Adirondacks she was relieved to see that Everit was greatly improved in health; in fact he seemed to shine with a new vitality and sense of purpose. The siblings had many things to discuss after their months apart. Everit told Kate that he would not have missed the hard experience he had endured, and that it helped him to better understand the suffering of others. He related an incident from his time in London: After dining one evening he went out for a walk; it was a cold night. He happened upon a group of poorly clad indigent men, huddled on the pavement in front of a Salvation Army mission. Something made him slow down and inquire about their situation. The men explained that they had nowhere to go and were waiting to claim a bed for the night. Everit hurried back to the comfort of his hotel but he could not erase the men's faces from his mind. He returned to the mission the next morning and was distressed to learn that the men were literally dumped from their cots at 5 a.m., given a cup of tea and a slice of bread, and turned back into the street.

This encounter opened Kate's brother's eyes to the suffering of the common man and gave him pause to consider the words of industrialist Andrew Carnegie as expressed in *The Gospel of Wealth*. First published in *The North American Review* in June 1898, Carnegie had written, "The problem of our age is the proper administration of wealth, so that the ties of brotherhood may still bind together the rich and poor in harmonious relationship." Everit agreed that it was essential for people of means to utilize their wealth in a thoughtful manner, a view very much in keeping with the Quaker philosophy that had guided generations of Macys. As he spoke, his words resonated with Kate; brother and sister began to consider how to use their fortunes to serve others. After a while Everit unexpectedly took on a lighter tone; he divulged details about his courtship and recent engagement to Miss Edith Wiseman Carpenter whose mother Josephine James Carpenter was well-known to Carrie. Edith and Everit had met in Europe and their courtship developed under the watchful eyes of their doting mothers. Everit presented his intended with a large and handsome pearl engagement ring set in gold. She was already busy planning a church wedding for February. Their nuptials would be followed by an elaborate Venetian-themed celebration. It was up to Everit to plan the honeymoon.

Kate was thrilled for Everit and his future bride, but her health continued to "run up and down." By November, when she and her Aunt Mary attended the wedding of Sarah Stillman and William Goodsell Rockefeller, the eldest son of longtime family friend William Avery Rockefeller, Mary Kingsland commented that Kate looked very frail, and she convinced her to return to Philadelphia to take what was called a partial rest cure. This meant that Kate would miss her brother's wedding.

Everit and Edith were married on February 18, 1896, at St. Bartholomew's Church in New York City. It was an extravagant affair with Edith's bridesmaids outfitted in matching tea length dresses. In her diary, Mary Kingsland commented on the beautiful music and the profusion of lilies and wrote, "I will never forget the tender look of love and perfect peace that shone on Everit's face, and I think that Edith equally felt the trust and love he reposed in her." The newlyweds visited Kate in Philadelphia before setting off on their adventurous honeymoon which began with a transcontinental train trip to San Francisco where they boarded a steamer bound for Yokohama, Japan. While in Japan Everit searched out Oriental art on the advice of his boyhood friend the artist Albert Herter who had also honeymooned in Japan. In this era Asian art and artifacts were all the rage. Everit maintained a meticulous record of each and every purchase made from Tokyo to Nagasaki, Kyoto, and Kobe; his avid interest in collecting began several years earlier when, as an architecture student at Columbia, he purchased an ancient Roman funerary cippus, a small marble tombstone from the Villa Borghese. The antiquity was shipped to Greystone, but overlooked during the tumultuous time of Mae's illness. It was all but lost and forgotten until 2015 when it was discovered during excavation work at the site of the modern Greystone development.

While the newlyweds experienced the Far East, Alaska, and the Canadian Rockies, Kate worked to regain her health in Philadelphia. It is difficult to know precisely how ill she was when Mary Kingsland had urged her to seek medical help the previous November. Perhaps Mary had overreacted showing an undue amount of concern about Kate as she continued to grieve over Mae.

By April, Walter, Kate, and Alice were back at the leased house in Morristown; they went up to Maine for the summer to avoid the heat that Kate found difficult to tolerate and stayed at her Cousin Carrol Macy's cottage in Bar Harbor. Carrie, who was nearby at an estate named Sea Urchin, was chronically under the weather and Kate felt concerned about her mother's overall well-being. However, she was unaware of the true nature of Carrie's ill-health. Rather than discuss it, her mother hid her suspected ailment and assured her daughter that she was suffering from her constant adversaries— rheumatism and arthritis—compounded by vagaries of encroaching old age (which may seem odd to the contemporary reader since she was not yet age sixty). Throughout that summer Kate counted Dr. Mitchell among her most devoted friends. He was a regular cottager on Mt. Desert Island, and even though he was not seeing patients he often walked up from his house on West Street for one of his helpful visits. During their intimate talks, Kate confided her concern about Carrie among other things. That fall, Mitchell convinced the Ladds to go to California for Kate's benefit, and Walter agreed. It is likely that he was aware that his mother-in-law had a serious illness and wished to protect his wife from the misery that was bound to come.

Chapter 21

KATE HAD ALWAYS DEPENDED ON WALTER TO TAKE A STAND and do what was best for her even when members of the Macy family criticized him for taking his wife away from the family. In the late 1890s, southern California seemed a world away from New York, and this may have been Dr. Mitchell's intention as he sought to protect Kate from family-related worries.

Kate, Walter, and Alice left the East Coast, after short stays at Morristown and New York, on November 24, 1896 and reached beautiful Pasadena by private car five days later. During the 1890s Pasadena was a most prosperous place. The community had more than doubled in size between the enumeration of the 1890 census and the year of the Ladds' arrival by which time Pasadena boasted about 12,000 residents.

The transplants spent a peaceful winter at the Hotel Green, which was the social center of Pasadena during the late nineteenth century and the winter home of some of the East Coast's most prominent industrialists. Throughout their stay in Pasadena Walter's activities were well documented in the local newspapers, which probably satisfied him immensely. He had never been acknowledged as a member of high society in the large pond of New York. In contrast, in his new locale, he could make a splash—Walter was viewed as an independently wealthy and sophisticated gentleman, a man whose actions were newsworthy in the budding city of Pasadena.

Since their arrival in Pasadena, Kate's health had improved so much that she and Walter decided to make it their permanent winter home. Walter rented the Orange Grove Avenue home of Mrs. Herbert C. Torrey on the Arroyo, with its wonderful view of the San Gabriel Mountains, and after fourteen years of marriage the Ladds purchased their first house from businessman John Wadsworth. The couple looked forward to taking occupancy of their home in the autumn after significant renovations were carried out.

The Wadsworth house, Colina Cottage, was designed by Frederick L. Roehrig, a Cornell-educated architect whose firm catered to those wealthy health seekers and businessmen who aspired to build showplaces in Southern California. Built in 1893 at a cost of $25,000, it was of eclectic design, uniting elements of both the American Craftsman and Shingle styles of architectures. Roehrig, who was called the Millionaire's Architect, was also known for his work on a number of Pasadena landmarks including the Hotel Green which like many of his distinctively designed residences is extant.

The Ladds' purchase of the Wadsworth property was major news; it warranted a full column of print in *The Los Angeles Times* on March 23, 1897.

> The largest real estate sale of the year was closed last Saturday morning. Walter G. Ladd of Morristown, New Jersey, purchased the beautiful place belonging to John Wadsworth on Columbia Street near Ocean Grove Avenue. There is no more desirable site in Pasadena. The house is at the summit of a hill, directly overlooking the arroyo and with a magnificent view of the city and mountains beyond. The property is considered one of the choicest spots for a home that Pasadena affords…Mr. Ladd came to Pasadena about last November and has been staying at the Hotel Green. He has traveled extensively in all parts of the world and came to Pasadena merely to spend the winter and without any intention of making it his home…"I knew nothing about Pasadena," said Mr. Ladd, "until I came here in November. I am surprised that it is not better known in the East. I have been charmed with the climate and the scenery. Nowhere in Switzerland nor in the Riviera have I seen more beautiful views…It is our intention to make this our winter home.

According to the newspaper the Ladds paid "in the neighborhood of $45,000 to $50,000" for their new home. In actuality they paid $41,250 for the place and renamed it "Vista Vasta" because as Kate recalled, it had one of the finest views in California.

With its magnificent setting, the house and three surrounding acres quickly commanded Walter's full attention. He enlarged his acreage with the purchase of additional parcels of land, expanded the size of the house, built a fine stable, and hired the prominent Scottish landscape architect Robert Gordon Fraser to bring his hillside to life, planting all manner of flora including sturdy young palms and fragrant citrus trees. A few years later Fraser would gain fame for transforming property along the Arroyo Seco into a garden unlike anything the West had ever seen when St. Louis beer baron Adolphus Busch commissioned him to design Busch Gardens.

Walter felt completely at home in Pasadena and commented that he was greatly pleased with the locality. With his fine home he became a founding member of the Pasadena Country Club, organized to "promote social intercourse among its members" and to encourage such outdoor sports such as golf.[1] As he eased his way into local society he continued to oversee "conspicuous improvements" on the house and grounds at 500 Columbia Street.[2]

While Walter maintained a public role, Kate and Alice remained behind the scenes and concentrated their energies on decorating the interior of Vista Vasta. Kate's furniture was sent out from New York and she and Alice redecorated every room; as Kate noted, it was exhausting work, but she and Alice had fun doing it. New York muralist Detleff Sammann was engaged to enhance the rooms of the house with his creative flair—his work was touted as an indulgence of the rich. Sammann was well-known among the connoisseurs of Europe as well as in New York where he maintained a studio. He was recognized as the greatest flower painter in America. His work was on display in both public buildings and private residences including such impressive locations as the Blue and Green Rooms of the White House, the library of the United States Capitol and at "Clayton," the Pittsburgh mansion of steel magnate Henry Clay Frick. *The Los Angeles Times* reported that Walter Ladd was one of Sammann's California patrons, surely a testament to his affluence and urbanity.[3]

Although the Ladds had relocated to Pasadena to benefit Kate's health, it seems that overall Walter gained more than she. Living thousands of miles from New York he was like a man reborn, able to reinvent himself and flaunt his wife's wealth; however, his affluent new associates perfunctorily assumed that he was a well-off man in his own right. They were impressed by his "conspicuous" and expensive additions to Vista Vasta as well as his commitment to his fragile wife. It appears that for Walter, life in Pasadena was like a dream come true: He owned one of the finest and most lavishly decorated homes in Southern California and was affiliated with a circle of wealthy and prominent men; he had achieved a dream that had long eluded him.

While Walter flourished, Kate's recently improved health was on the wane. During the spring and summer of 1897 she repeatedly received tragic news from home that affected her overall state of well-being: First, she learned of the death of her Aunt Cornelia Macy Walker. She was Josiah's sister, the quiet and devoted Macy daughter who rarely strayed far from her mother Eliza's side. Far more shocking and difficult for Kate to comprehend was the news of the death of five-year-old Valentine Willets, Mae and Howard's youngest boy. Little was communicated about the nature of his death but Kate believed that an accident had caused it. Kate's heart ached, especially for her mother and Val's older brothers Jack and Josiah, and she longed to be of comfort to them. She surrounded herself with her nephews' photographs; among them was a recent portrait of little Valentine. Dressed in a sailor suit, blonde hair crowned by a beribboned straw hat, his face exuded an innocence so pure that as she clung to the image, Kate could not help but weep for her sister Mae. Years later, she reported that it had been a hot and dry summer throughout which she suffered from insomnia which plagued her for the duration of her time in California.

It is likely that Kate felt conflicted about remaining in Pasadena during the summer of 1897. While Alice and Walter made several trips east between 1897 and 1898, she never joined them—she was continually discouraged from travel, ostensibly because the journey might take a toll of her health. In reality, she was dissuaded from travel for a different reason. Unbeknown to Kate, her mother was seriously ill with breast cancer. Carrie Macy underwent surgery late in the spring of 1897, probably in Bar Harbor, where she had taken out a long-term lease on Steepways Cottage on the Cleftstone Road. Kate's family kept her in the dark intentionally, fearing that she would insist upon returning home to care for her mother as she had done for Mae, and seriously compromise her health.

Throughout her time in Pasadena, Kate also missed opportunities to attend the happy family occasions that always brought her joy. As she and Alice put the finishing touches on the house, in the fall of 1897, she missed the celebration of Mary and William Kingsland's Golden Wedding Anniversary. Kate may have been puzzled to learn that Carrie did not attend either, but she probably assumed that her mother's absence was related to the recent death of Valentine Willets, not because she was recuperating from cancer surgery. Mother and daughter both regretted not being part of the Kingslands' unique occasion and they sent telegrams, flowers, and gifts of solid gold. Mary Kingsland relayed the news that a great deal of champagne was served; her husband had spared no expense. To commemorate the occasion he presented his wife of fifty years with a gold coffee service made by the Tiffany Company of Newark, New Jersey and he further sought to commemorate the milestone anniversary by commissioning a pair of oil portraits to be rendered by the world famous Spanish artist Raimundo de Madrazzo y Garretta.

It is difficult to know how Kate passed her time in Pasadena. She enjoyed the weather, especially the balmy days of winter, as well as the change of scenery, but it does not appear that she joined local society as Walter did. Much of her time between the summer of 1897 and the end of 1898 was spent quietly with Alice, often behind closed doors. She felt adrift without her wide group of friends and family who had always played an important role in her life.

New Year's Day 1899 began with rain tapping at Kate's window causing her to question whether the inclement weather would affect the viewing of the Tenth Annual Tournament of Roses Parade which had been the talk of the town for months. It was expected that crowds would usher in the new year by gathering to watch garland-covered carriages amble through downtown but as the unusually foul weather persisted, the long-awaited festivities were cancelled. Perhaps Kate and Alice passed the morning quietly at home, putting away Christmas ornaments, working on a new jigsaw puzzle, or sewing contentedly in the parlor. In Kate's mind, Alice could always turn even the stormiest day into a sunny one with her pleasant chatter and easy laugh. At some point, however, they were interrupted: A Western Union messenger boy appeared with a telegram, which announced that sixty-year-old Carrie Macy had died at 11:30 p.m. the previous evening. Kate was thunderstruck because she said that she was not aware that her mother had been seriously ill. The final two months of Carrie's life had been dire. The Kingslands were so devastated that they could not even bring themselves to record the loss of the sister-in-law whom they called sister in their diaries. Belatedly, Kate learned that her mother had been ill for some time—

as she turned past events over in her mind it all began to make sense. She remembered that Carrie had been nursing a sore arm while in France and she had settled in Bar Harbor in early spring and remained far beyond the close of the season. Overcome by grief, Kate felt tremendous remorse over her prolonged separation from her mother. Even though she knew that her family sought to spare her worry, she was incensed that she had been denied the opportunity to tell her mother goodbye. Carrie was buried in the Macy family plot at Woodlawn on January 3, 1899, joining her husband in peaceful repose after more than twenty-three lonely years as a widow.

Dressed in mourning garb, Kate drifted about the rooms of the magnificent Vista Vasta feeling as homesick as a child. She made her need to go home abundantly clear to Walter. He acquiesced with the belief that they would resume residence in Pasadena the following winter. Nonetheless, even though the Ladds held on to Vista Vasta for the next eight years they never returned to California. On January 27, 1907 the *Los Angeles Herald* would report, "A tract measuring 1650 feet on Columbia Avenue was sold by the Walter G. Ladd estate to C.W. Gates for $80,000." Charles Warner Gates was a Midwestern-born lumberman, and even though the Ladds were handsomely paid for Vista Vasta, Walter struggled over the decision to relinquish his liberated life in the West.

Chapter 22

BEFORE MOVING EAST, HOWEVER, WALTER ENJOYED what would be his last hurrah in Pasadena society when he presented a valuable sterling silver loving cup to John S. Cravens, the winner of a three-day golf tournament played at the Pasadena Country Club. *The Los Angeles Times* mentioned Walter Ladd by name and reported, "Golf that delighted the experts was seen during this match."[1] Shortly thereafter, he, Kate, and Alice made their way to New York returning by private car just as they had arrived in California two and a half years earlier. They spent the remainder of the year in Lenox, Massachusetts, and in the winter of 1900 moved on to Tuxedo, New York where Kate said that she was ill for the entire time. It is likely that she felt guilt-ridden and depressed over her mother's death throughout this period.

One way that Kate coped with her sadness, grief, and physical illness was by trying to do something for others. We are reminded of the thirteen-year-old who so desperately wished to read to the infirm to mitigate the pain she felt after the death of her father. Even as a girl, Kate understood that she could gain strength and resilience when she ignored her own despair and focused on helping someone else. As an adult woman with independent means she learned that engagement with significant charitable endeavors could add greater purpose to her life, an insight that paved the way for the philanthropy that would come to define her.

Edward Trudeau was a health crusader without equal in his day, known for his pioneering work with tuberculosis (TB). It is likely that he had opened Kate's eyes to the need for private financial support for convalescence and medical research, areas that would one day be the focus of her philanthropic activity and provide her with opportunities to put the needs of strangers before her own.

Throughout Kate's lifetime tuberculosis was a terrifying illness, recognized by many names including "consumption," "the captain of death," and "the white plague" (a reference to the anemic pallor that characterized sufferers). From the nineteenth century through the early years of the twentieth century tuberculosis was the leading cause of death in the United States; at the dawn of the twentieth century 400 Americans lost their lives to the disease daily.[2] European immigrants and African Americans were disproportionally affected by the ailment, but it also brought premature death to comfortably well-off Americans including Kate's beloved childhood friend Sallie Whitcomb Sterling, who lingered in a sanitarium near Morristown before she died at the age of thirty. It was not until the late 1940s that researchers would finally discover a pharmaceutical cure for "the white plague."[3]

In 1872, Edward Trudeau, by then a New York City physician, husband, and father was diagnosed with tuberculosis, universally called consumption. He knew it was likely a death sentence; Edward had nursed his older brother Francis throughout the darkest days of his ordeal with consumption. Francis did not survive. Faced with the distinct possibility of an early death, Trudeau left his wife Charlotte and their two small children to seek a cure. Following an unsuccessful stint in the warmer environs of South Carolina, he traveled to the Adirondacks in upstate New York where he stayed at the St. Regis Lake House also known as Paul Smith's Hotel; the hostelry primarily catered to well-heeled sportsmen. Trudeau's health temporarily improved in the mountain air; however, he suffered a serious relapse when he resumed city life. He was advised to go to Minnesota for further exposure to fresh air and sunshine; this time his family accompanied him, but his health did not pick up, leading the Trudeaus to come home and settle at Paul Smith's for the summer of 1874. They extended their stay through the following winter. Throughout those long isolated months the Trudeaus relied upon Paul and Lydia Smith and their sons, the only full-time residents of St. Regis Lake. The family saw to their daily needs and their comfort and companionship must have been a godsend. Feeling the benefit of the bracing environment Trudeau decided to spend the following winter in a leased house in the village of Saranac Lake. Propelled by the belief that an exposure to fresh air was key to curing consumption, the Trudeaus decided to stay in the Adirondacks year-round.[4] Although his wife Charlotte Beare Trudeau was a refined woman with a preference for city life, her devotion to her husband never wavered. She remained by her husband's side until his death in 1915. It seems likely that without a wife of Charlotte Trudeau's disposition, Edward Trudeau might have remained in New York City to face an early and excruciating death.[5]

By the winter of 1877-78 an increasing number of well-off consumptives began to join the Trudeaus and embrace a commitment to an outdoor way of life. Trudeau's physician and friend, Dr. Alfred Loomis, is credited with persuading pulmonary patients of the positive health effect of wintering in the Adirondacks.

Trudeau's personal experience convinced him of the need to develop an effective course of treatment for his fellow sufferers. In 1884, with the financial help of wealthy patrons, he established the first American sanitarium and research facility dedicated to the study of pulmonary disease. The Adirondack Cottage Sanitarium at Saranac Lake was established to treat individuals who could not otherwise afford to convalesce in the fresh mountain air.[6] Trudeau's work was based in part on the groundbreaking efforts of two other men: Dr. Hermann Brehmann and Dr. Robert Koch. Brehmann was a Silesian physician and botanist who, like Trudeau suffered from tuberculosis. He found that his medical condition improved while studying plant life in the Himalayas; this inspired him to establish a hospital, which became a model for the treatment of consumptives throughout Europe. Trudeau was further influenced by the research findings of Dr. Robert Koch who, in 1882, confirmed that tuberculosis was a contagious disease caused by a specific germ: tubercle bacillus.

Trudeau built his sanitarium on a well-protected hillside less than one mile from the village of Saranac Lake; he designed an enclave of intimate patient homes meant to recreate the ambiance of a pleasant residential village. The community consisted of "twenty wooden, brick, or stone cottages, given by wealthy patrons, designed usually for four patients, each having a separate room, and so arranged that each room opens on a spacious, sunny, but well-protected veranda, upon which a bed may be rolled."[7] Advocates of the cottage plan stressed that the home-like nature of the arrangement benefited patients who might spend years away from home. In addition, the smaller scale design helped to mitigate the risk of reinfection within the patient community. When possible, Trudeau hired doctors and nurses who had themselves recovered from tuberculosis; he believed that survivors of the disease were better equipped to understand the difficulties that his patients endured.

As we have learned, Kate probably became aware of Trudeau's pioneering work in 1895 when she and Walter spent the summer in the Adirondacks at the Cooper camp. Thereafter, she was stimulated to join other wealthy New Yorkers, including her mother, who offered Trudeau financial support. They provided money as well as donations of items to be sold at the sanitarium's annual fundraiser which was initiated by Helen Stokes in 1884.[8] Among Trudeau's most dependable New York City supporters were Mrs. Stokes and her husband Anson Phelps Stokes, Elizabeth Milbank Anderson, and George Campbell Cooper. Cooper funded Trudeau's original laboratory with a gift of $10,000; after an 1894 fire completely destroyed the lab, public health philanthropist Elizabeth Milbank

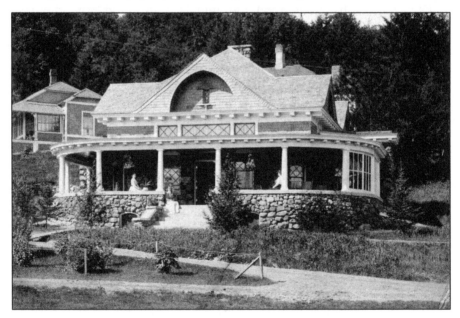

Ladd Cottage *(The Adirondack Collection, Saranac Lake Free Library, Saranac Lake, NY)*

Anderson stepped in to provide funds to rebuild and expand the facility which, became known as the Saranac Laboratory for the Study of Tuberculosis.[9]

Throughout the summer of 1899, as Kate grappled with her health she thought often of her sister and considered how she might honor Mae's memory in a lasting and constructive way. After considering several options, she asked Walter to contact Dr. Trudeau to discuss funding a new patient cottage at Saranac as a permanent memorial to her sister. Even though it was meant as a tribute to Mae Macy Willets, the place was always called "Ladd Cottage."[10]

Walter functioned as Kate's representative on the project, corresponding with Dr. Trudeau for more than a year to review costs and ensure that everything was done according to his wife's specifications. His initial letter sheds further light on Kate's thinking,

> My dear Dr. Trudeau,
>
> Mrs. Milbank has already informed you of our Enquiry as to whether there is a need of a cottage at the A.C.S...Mrs. Ladd has been thinking of establishing a free bed in some New York Hospital in memory of her sister but as we are interested in your sanitarium we have thought the same purpose could be accomplished by building a cottage. I enclose a draft of a letter, which if you approve and will return to me I will have prepared and on acceptance of the offer by the Trustees the money will be forthcoming.[11]

He concluded his message "with pleasant remembrances of your kindness in the past..."

A week later Walter followed up with a letter to the trustees of the Adirondack Cottage Sanitarium: "I am requested by Mrs. Ladd to offer you on her account the sum of $7,500.00..." The letter stipulated that at least $4,000 of Kate's donation was to be dedicated to building and furnishing a cottage for patients and that "a tablet be set and maintained in some suitable place in said cottage bearing an inscription to the effect that the cottage has been built in memory of Mary Kingsland Macy Willets by her sister Mrs. Walter Graeme Ladd, 1899."[12]

Further review of the correspondence between Walter and Dr. Trudeau makes it clear that Walter was as acutely involved in the details regarding the erection of the building at Saranac as he had been in developing the grounds at Vista Vasta in Pasadena. His letters, written between August 1899 and October, 1900, provide us with a glimpse into a man who liked to manage things. His vigilance was important because Kate held high expectations for the quality of the cottage and its furnishings.

The shingle-style dwelling was designed by New York architect William L. Coulter, a pulmonary patient, who was responsible for the design of five endowed cottages at the sanitarium. In early September Coulter sent Walter a detailed description of the proposed project and anticipated costs. By all accounts Ladd cottage was the most elaborate of the patient cottages.[13] The structure was wood-framed with a cobble-stone veneer. It stood one and one-half stories tall and was equipped with multiple bathrooms, closets, chestnut and oak woodwork, bronze hardware, and an outdoor sleeping porch which typified the patient cottage plan. To further memorialize Mae, the Ladds commissioned the Tiffany Glass and Decorating Company to design a bronze plaque in her name, intended for display in the cottage's center hall. Ladd Cottage was purportedly the most expensive of the Adirondack Cottage Sanitarium patient homes; ultimately, Kate spent in excess of $8,500 (or more than $200,000 in today's money) to fully outfit and maintain it.[14] Some twenty-eight years later, sanitarium superintendent C.R. Armstrong described Ladd Cottage as "one of our finest" and the one "most often shown to visitors."[15]

Chapter 23

Bar Harbor, Maine

June 18, 1900

My dear Doctor Trudeau,

Your favor of the 20th ulto. came safely to hand and I should have written ere this but for the fact that owing to Mrs. Ladd's health I have not felt equal to writing letters: this you will readily appreciate when I tell you that it was found necessary to operate on Mrs. Ladd on the 22nd ulto. for the removal of a tumor from her left breast.[1] We were fortunate to be able to have Dr. Abbe operate and I am thankful to be able to say that the operation was a success from a surgical point of view and the examination of the proteins removed show that the operation was an "Early one" and we are assured that we need not fear a recurrence of the tumor; also that while it is was not a malignant tumor at the stage it had attained, yet if it had not been removed the end would have been inevitable. We have also been fortunate in having Dr. Schley with us to care for Mrs. Ladd—he is an assistant of Dr. Abbe—able and a most pleasant personality. We hope to be able to keep him with us until the wound is entirely healed and Mrs. Ladd well on the road to health. Unfortunately, Mrs. Ladd has suffered much of late from rheumatism and neuralgia and besides from being distressful this has doubtless retarded the progress of the wound somewhat: however, though slow, her progress is entirely satisfactory. We have only advised a few intimate friends of the operation so it is probably not generally known.[2]

After enduring months of pain associated with a combination of rheumatism and neuralgia, thirty-seven-year-old Kate made the gut-wrenching discovery of a small lump in her breast. Typically, women felt so paralyzed by fear when faced with the possibility of breast cancer that they did nothing. But, unlike most women, Kate had a good deal of personal experience with the disease that had carried a death sentence for her sister and her mother. She consulted a doctor right away and was advised to undergo a mastectomy without delay.

Kate later recalled, "In the Spring of 1900, Dr. Abbe was called and
he said my breast must be removed. So after we were moved to Bar
Harbor, he performed the operation at Elsinore, the place now owned
by Mrs. Dimock. I nearly died and was left a perfect wreck from the
operation."[3]

Kate's surgeon, Dr. Robert Waldo Abbe, was a New York City-
born physician and a man of diverse interests and abilities. He was an
eminent surgeon who made numerous contributions to his profession,
particularly in the fields of vascular and reconstructive surgery and
cancer treatment. A colleague of French scientists Marie and Pierre
Curie, Abbe was the first American doctor to use radium; he is
considered the founder of the field of radiation therapy in the United
States.[4]

Two months before performing Kate's mastectomy the doctor
presented a paper to the New York Academy of Medicine at a
meeting devoted to the topic of cancer of the breast. He told his
colleagues that "Cancer of the breast should be caught at its birth and
eradicated then and there," and he encouraged his audience to perform
mastectomies, describing the removal of a woman's breast as "a
practically bloodless operation," stating that a radical approach
guaranteed a nonrecurrence in the breast wall because there was
"nothing left in which the cancer could return." Abbe advocated the
complete removal of the afflicted breast, as well as a large area of
skin, fat, glands, and pectoral muscle to confer immunity from further
recurrence.[5]

Twenty-first century advances in the understanding and treatment
of breast cancer would have seemed unfathomable to Kate and the
medical men of the time. In 1900, some physicians persisted in
blaming a woman for her condition; they called breast cancer a
"female malady" akin to menstrual irregularities and, therefore, the
product of a diseased mind.[6] Sir James Paget, the preeminent mid-
nineteenth century British cancer authority stated, "The cases are so
frequent in which deep anxiety, deferred hope, and disappointment,
are quickly followed by the growth or increase of cancer that we can
hardly doubt that mental depression is a weighty addition to the other
influences that favour the development of the cancerous
constitution."[7]

Women's experiences with breast cancer have been documented

for centuries, and although Kate's mastectomy was traumatic, she was far more fortunate than those who came before her. Influenced by William Stewart Halstead, whose radical mastectomy was the gold standard in breast cancer treatment through the 1960s, Dr. Abbe employed exacting surgical techniques based on the best medical knowledge available. He followed Joseph Lister's aseptic techniques and made his patients more comfortable through the use of anesthesia. When combined with early detection and immediate action, these practices provided somewhat improved women's outcomes. Despite these improvements, in 1900 less than twenty percent of women survived more than five years post-surgery. We recall that Kate's sister Mae languished for one year after her mastectomy; her mother Carrie survived for eighteen months.

By all accounts, into the nineteenth century, mastectomies were atavistic interventions—bloody, crude, and dehumanizing operations undertaken in unsanitary environments. In one documented instance a woman's breast was held by large fishhook lances attached to ropes— her surgeon pulled on the ropes to lift the breast off the chest wall, cut her flesh with a large knife, and cauterized the bleeding with hot irons.[8] This patient would have endured her surgery strapped to a chair, one arm held firmly above her head by the doctor's male assistant. Prior to the advent of ether, circa 1846, she faced the knife fully awake and was expected to remain calm and stoic throughout her ordeal of twenty-five to thirty minutes. A surgeon's speed was essential and at best, the terrified patient may have been offered a cordial beforehand to calm her nerves. A particularly harrowing description of breast removal is offered through the experience of Abigail Adams Smith, the only daughter of President John Adams and his wife. Mrs. Smith faced breast cancer surgery in 1811. At the age of forty-two she had discovered a lump in her breast but waited for two years before consulting with noted Philadelphia physician Benjamin Rush. He advised that there should be no delay in "flying to the knife."[9] Abigail Smith's mastectomy was performed by Dr. John Warren in a bedroom at the Adams's home in Quincy, Massachusetts. The ill woman was seated and restrained. Her surgeon straddled her body; his surgical instruments were limited to a large fork with two finely sharpened prongs and a wooden handled razor. When Mrs. Smith's breast was separated from her chest, the doctor used the fork to lift it away and proceeded to use the razor to attack tumors that had formed under her arm. Abigail's wounds were cauterized with a red hot spatula, then crudely sutured and bandaged. She was awake throughout the entire procedure. The woman maintained faith that her horrific ordeal would cure her. Sadly, this was not the case; after a brief rally, Abigail Adams Smith fell desperately ill. Her well-known father cared for her until she died, less than one year post-surgery.[10]

Although Kate felt indebted to Abbe and his assistant Scott Schley for their care, Phoebe Edgar, the secretary who helped Kate prepare her memoir, described her employer's state of mind and concerns before and after the surgery,

> Dr. Robert Abbe did a very extensive operation and she had a perfectly frightful time. Naturally, she had a picture in her mind of repeating her sister's long and horrible death. Dr. Abbe was a surgeon and nothing else—he understood nothing of her nervous system and he terrified her. He told her he had done a grand job but she had the other breast to consider and watch very carefully and avoid knocks or the slightest injuries. Mrs. Ladd was several years getting over the operation.[11]

Viewed more than a century later, Abbe's remarks reflect a lack of compassion for his female cancer patients. Like most of his fellow practitioners, Abbe was focused on achieving an exacting and complete amputation and failed to acknowledge the psychological consequences of breast cancer.

It is possible that Walter was unaware of the psychological effects of his wife's illness as well. One month post-surgery, he wrote Dr. Trudeau that her progress was slow but satisfactory. He was concerned about her recovery but confident that she was in good hands with Dr. Schley who was in residence for the summer and this may have led him to underplay the precarious nature of her state of health, especially when he went out into society.

While Kate clung to life in the privacy of Elsinore, the Bar Harbor season was in high gear. Golfers, male and female alike, hit the links at the Kebo Valley Club where they took lessons from the well-known Scotish professional James Douglass. Yacht racing was in full force and preparations for the annual horse show and summer fair were underway. The doyennes of society entertained guests at teas, luncheons, and dinner parties. The Jordan Pond House, a popular gathering spot for both "the angler and the lover of picturesque hill scenery" was abuzz once more.[12] *The New York Times* disclosed that "Dr. W.S. Schley, son of Admiral Schley, is spending the season with the Ladds at Elsinore, Hugh McMillan's beautiful place on the heights, near Green Mountain."[13]

The newspaper society column offers no hint as to the reason behind Schley's stay at Elsinore. Members of the summer colony may have assumed that the young doctor was a New York friend of Mr. and Mrs. Walter Ladd, a man in need of a change of scenery. His status as a guest rather than as a physician helped to protect the Ladds' privacy at a time when a diagnosis of breast cancer was not discussed outside a woman's small close circle. As Walter had indicated to Dr. Trudeau, his wife's condition was only known by "a few intimate friends." While it was expected that the twenty-seven-year-old Dr. Schley would oversee the healing of Kate's wound, he also provided much-needed companionship to Walter. The men were guests at a variety of social events including a lawn reception and musicale for more than one hundred people at Westover, the summer home of Schley's friends Mr. and Mrs. Henry Lane Eno.[14] Ultimately, it was Alice Lemley who remained by Kate's side, and provided both the nursing care and the emotional support so critical to her recovery.

Kate's brother Everit and his wife Edith also provided support when they visited Bar Harbor. Even though he was a young man, Everit was no stranger to the ravages of breast cancer; he had been closely involved in the care of both his sister Mae and his mother during the most difficult days of their illnesses. Significantly, thirteen years later, he and Edith would join a committee of physicians and laypeople charged with establishing an organization to fight cancer, the result of which was the creation of "The American Society for the Control of Cancer," the forerunner of the American Cancer Society. The organization called attention to breast cancer by launching a public health campaign to encourage all women to consult a physician at the first sign of a breast lump. It was known that early detection was critical to survival; the organization maintained that surgery was the only cure. As a result, between 1905 and 1925, the number of cancer surgeries performed in the United States steadily rose. This was accompanied by a slow but steady increase in survival rates.

Chapter 24

AFTER SPENDING SEVERAL MONTHS IN SECLUSION AT ELSINORE, Kate returned to New York City, hoping that better days were ahead. She, Walter, and Alice lived on Riverside Drive near her cousin George.

That winter, Kate's optimism was dashed and her precarious state of health was further compromised when a dentist inadvertently broke her jaw during a tooth extraction. As a result, she was limited to an all liquid diet for nine months. As Kate sought to rebuild her body and spirit she faced further personal sadness when her grandmother Eliza Macy, Uncle Silvanus, and beloved nephew Jack Willets all passed away within quick succession. While she mourned the passing of her Macy relatives, they had enjoyed long, wonderful lives. In contrast, her sister's firstborn died at the age of seventeen. Kate commented that he was like her own child, "his going was a great blow to me."[1] She was further dismayed to learned that her beloved sister-in-law Rebe Ladd had been hospitalized with nervous distress. Kate had but few details regarding her condition; however, she was comforted to know that her niece Frances was safely under the care of the Serrills in Darby, Pennsylvania.

Compounding these sorrows was a growing conflict within the four walls of her own home concerning Alice Lemley. Simply put, Walter did not care for Alice. He felt that she did nothing constructive, had outgrown her usefulness, and should be dismissed. Kate struggled with how best to deflect Walter's baseless insinuations about her companion and dearest friend. She told Walter unequivocally that Alice's unconditional love and dependable nursing care were vital to her recovery and continued happiness. To the outside world, "Miss Lemley" was Kate's loyal nurse and companion. To Kate, her "Chick-a-Dee" would always be one of her greatest blessings and the person who meant everything to her.[2]

Within the pages of her memoir, Kate has inserted an unexpected and haunting image, a photograph from this unsettled period. Perhaps it is her way of telling us that, despite having reached her lowest ebb, this dark interlude signified an important turning point in her life. An unknown photographer, poised behind a tripod-mounted camera has

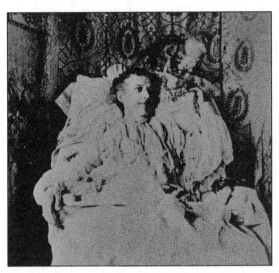

Kate, age 39 *(From her personal memoir, The Story of My Life)*

managed to poignantly capture the essence of Kate Macy Ladd's enduring faith and resilience. It is 1902, and Kate is two years post-cancer surgery; she has just endured another surgical procedure. She describes herself as a great invalid and comments that while the operation to remove an unspecified growth was not serious it "added to deplete me."[3] She weighs a staggering seventy-two pounds and her hair is sparse and tinged with grey. We look at her emaciated face, searching for a familiar trace, and for a moment it is difficult to *find* Kate; it would be easy to mistake her for one of Dr. Trudeau's most ravaged consumptives. She is propped up in bed surrounded by a mass of white linen and a three-sided quilted screen. Closer scrutiny reveals her to be tranquil and composed, and her serious, dark eyes reflect her resolute will to live.

During this bleak period, Kate thought about how difficult it would be for a woman with limited resources to recover from surgery, illness, or emotional despair. She recognized that the combination of her personal experience and wealth placed her in a unique position to help other women to recuperate with comfort and dignity. Alice and Kate discussed this concept, and they began to hatch a plan aimed at improving women's lives. As Kate convalesced under Alice's attentive care, the women talked about the possibility of establishing a private convalescent home where women with limited means would be welcomed without charge. They envisioned a place where a woman's body and spirit would be uplifted in a supportive community. Years later, Kate remembered that she had thought about this throughout her "sick hard years," and it seems likely that her focus on helping other women contributed to her own recovery.[4]

Even though Kate was exceedingly frail, she and Walter continued to follow a nomadic path, migrating between Bar Harbor and New York City where they leased a fashionable townhouse next to family friends John D. Rockefeller, Jr. and his wife Abby Aldrich. Her father's one-time Standard Oil partner, John D. Rockefeller, Sr., also lived close by. Despite her pleasant situation Kate longed to put down permanent roots in a home of her own where she and Alice could realize their dream of a women's convalescent home.

As she approached her fortieth birthday, Kate recognized that she was a practical woman; we see no lingering sign of the innocent girl who was swept off her feet by a handsome stranger at Richfield Springs. Nevertheless, time and illness had taken a toll on Kate, and she was cut to the quick by those who vocalized the suspicion that Walter had married her for her money. She would never admit that at age eighteen she had been too young and inexperienced to accurately weigh Walter's merits and flaws; as a result, she spent her life declaring that he was a model husband, loyal and dependable. In 1903, the Ladds were poised to celebrate their twentieth wedding anniversary. Although their relationship was more businesslike than romantic, Kate never forgot how Walter had attended to her needs early in their marriage—he visited her day and night when she stayed at the Lexington Sanitarium and he was always willing to travel to engage the best doctors to care for her. More recently, Walter had relinquished a life that suited him well in Pasadena so that Kate could live in closer proximity to her family. Once the couple resettled in the east, he saw that Mae's memorial cottage at Saranac was built according to his wife's instructions, and it was Walter who made the arrangements for Kate's surgery and convalescence at Elsinore.

Over the course of her marriage, Kate had inherited a small fortune from the estates of her parents and grandparents. Notwithstanding the tenuous nature of Walter and Carrie's relationship, she had always assumed that her mother would remember her husband in her will so that he would have his own income. However, when Carrie Macy's will was probated, Kate was stunned to learn that her mother, whose property was worth over one and a half million dollars, did not bequeath Walter a single penny. Kate felt tremendously hurt by her mother's slight.[5] Without an income of his own, Walter remained wholly dependent upon his wife's money, which made him a kept man and, in his era, less of a man.

Walter's untenable position intensified once the Ladds lived in the vicinity of New York where gossip concerning Walter's "lack of suitability" persisted and created a difficult state of affairs for both husband and wife. To counteract this difficulty, Kate and Walter struck a bargain. Alice Lemley would remain a member of the Ladd household, and Walter would receive his own money from Kate's annual income. The arrangement allowed Kate to continue her practice of giving generous gifts and make charitable donations as she saw fit; once these personal expenses were covered all of her excess annual income was turned over to Walter to manage her financial affairs. Under the agreement, Walter paid for all household, medical, and travel expenses as well as costs associated with the building, furnishing, and landscaping of any future homes. Once these obligations were met Walter was "given all excess surplus." In other words, the leftover money belonged to him, and he had carte blanche to use it as he wished.[6]

With their agreement in force the Ladds decided to build homes near New York City and Bar Harbor: Walter may have been reluctant to settle in Westchester, New York, where so many Macys held country seats and where Kate's brother was planning to locate a country place near the Kingsland estate on the Hudson. Since the Ladds were favorably disposed to the area around Morristown, New Jersey, they returned to the vicinity to get a better sense of the lay of the land and leased two prominent properties successively. The first was Overcross, the Haley Fiske estate in the Bernardsville Mountain Colony. It was followed by Overleigh, the John Milton Dillon place in Far Hills. Overleigh, said to be one of the most attractive mansions in the Somerset Hills, was located on the main thoroughfare to Bernardsville; from this vantage point Walter could work with a broker and investigate properties that came up for sale. He also had begun to explore the purchase of a well-situated parcel of land for a second home at Bar Harbor. In the summer of 1904, he and Kate chartered the houseboat *Thetis* and he searched for a suitable water-front property where he planned to build a summer home. By then Kate's weight had increased slightly; even though she weighed less than ninety pounds, she had gained enough strength to walk with assistance. Years later, Kate reminisced that once she moved to New Jersey, her strength and energy began to soar and claimed that she was capable of accomplishing more in a day than most people. Her secretary Miss Edgar concurred, explaining that when she was feeling well, Kate had tremendous drive and would tire out two or three companions. Nonetheless, she was known to go "too hard" and then suffer the consequences.[7]

In April 1905, with the assistance of estate agents Nicholas and Lumis, the Ladds began to make land acquisitions in what would become Peapack-Gladstone, Far Hills, and Bedminster. They quickly purchased 560 acres. Within a few years the couple had amassed one of the largest estates in the Somerset Hills, encompassing almost 1,000 acres.[8] Kate and Walter chose a somewhat mysterious name for their estate: "Natirar"—an anagram for "Raritan," in recognition of the bubbling North Branch of the Raritan River that meandered for some two miles through the property. Perhaps Kate acknowledged that the 1903 "agreement" was working well—Walter's ability to assemble such an extensive property all but guaranteed that she and Alice would find an agreeable spot for the establishment of a convalescent home somewhere on the grounds of their property.

During this period, Walter strengthened ties with his brothers William, Henry, and Jim. Their elderly father William Whitehead Ladd, Sr. had just passed away after spending years under Henry's roof in Rutherford, New Jersey where he was the minister at Grace Church. Of all the Ladds, Walter and Kate had always been closest with Jim and Rebe; Kate was especially fond of their only daughter Frances whom she liked to treat with special gifts on birthdays and holidays. She and Walter also helped Jim and Rebe purchase a handsome home in Ardmore, Pennsylvania, on the train line to Philadelphia where Jim worked as a mechanical engineer. Kate believed that it was important to provide for other Ladd relatives, and she did so against Walter's wishes—he was known to speak derisively of William and Henry's children and said he had no interest in them. Nevertheless, Kate persisted in showing them kindness; it was her nature.

If Walter had been well-versed about the historical significance of his newly acquired land in the Somerset Hills, he may have enjoyed the opportunity to regale his less affluent brothers with details of his property's unique history. The native people of New Jersey were members of the Lenni-Lenape tribe. Notably, "Peapack" is derived from a Lenni-Lenape word for "place of water roots." The land that formed the core of Natirar was part of the historic Peapack Patent, more than 10,000 acres of prime land once in the possession of the Proprietors of the Province of New Jersey. The Patent was so expansive that it covered what would become the boroughs of Peapack and Gladstone as well as much of the future Bedminster Township. One of the first "improved" roads in the vicinity, the Peapack Path, crossed the property in the early 1730s, winding along an ancient Native American trail.[9]

Over the course of the eighteenth and nineteenth centuries the land was divided up and changed hands many times. A portion of the Peapack Patent had passed on to the American Revolutionary War General William Alexander, the self-styled "Lord Stirling," who also maintained a vast family estate nearby in Basking Ridge. In 1766 he sold his 900-acre parcel of the Peapack Patent to James Parker, a loyalist and prominent citizen of Perth Amboy. Parker, who never occupied the property, hired an agent to oversee it, and in 1801 his widow sold a large parcel of land to Nicholas Arrowsmith (or Arrosmith). A short time later, a small section, "Lot No. 2" of the original Peapack Patent, was conveyed to brothers-in-law Gilbert Lane and Abraham Nevius who initially worked their 186-acre lot as partners. Nevertheless, when the men further divided the lot Nevius retained a ninety-five-acre stake which remained in his family for more than ninety years.

Vestiges of the Nevius family settlement, such as barns and outbuildings, were evident when the Ladds acquired the property. Early in his tenure, Nevius had set up a saw mill powered by a stream on the property to produce lumber for the construction of barns on his farmstead. By the late 1850s the farm had been passed to Nevius's son-in-law, John Rodman. Rodman, known to be a man of means, did not immediately settle on the farm; however, he is credited with making multiple improvements to the property that made the place seem "entirely new." The farm passed on to Reverend Abraham Nevius Wyckoff and his sister Mary who lived there until 1895.[10]

Had he discussed the history of his estate, Walter may have referred to November 1895 as the start of the modern era of the property, for this was when Zachariah Belcher IV and his wife Kate Fuller acquired the Nevius-Rodman farm. The couple called their country home Sunnybranch Farm and resided there for a decade before selling their 200-acre portion of the historic Peapack Patent to the Ladds.

Zachariah Belcher was the treasurer of the Watts Campbell Company, a manufacturer of steam engines similar to the massive Corliss Engine that had powered the 1876 Centennial Exposition that Kate recalled from her youth. Once the Belchers took over the former Nevius-Rodman farm, they transformed it, building a new house on a ridge behind the barns. Belcher had a talent for growing flowers and carefully tended the landscape. Locals assumed that the Belchers were content at Sunnybranch Farm. Therefore, some neighbors may have been surprised to learn that the property had been conveyed to the Ladds. It is reasonable to assume that Walter was in a position to pay

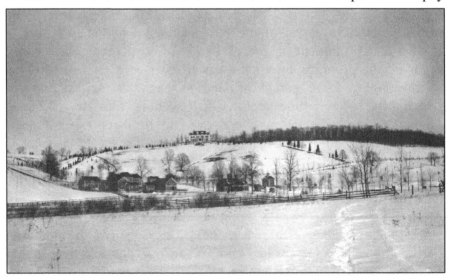

Sunnybranch Farm, circa 1905, by Fred Pitney Crater *(Courtesy of the Bernardsville Public Library Local History Collection, Bernardsville, NJ)*

for it handsomely. That the Belchers were happy in the area is borne
out by their subsequent move. With Ladd's money they purchased
another piece of property nearby and called it Lo-An-Oak Farm.
There they renovated an old farmhouse into a twenty-room mansion
and surrounded it with lush lawns and gardens. It was said that they
added a music room with perfect acoustics.

Between 1905 and 1912, Walter was busy attending to the details
of his two future homes, a mansion on the Natirar property as well as
a sizable house on a parcel that he had acquired at Sonogee Point on
Frenchman's Bay. The Ladds would follow their anagram naming
practice and call their summer home "Eegonos," the reverse of
Sonogee. The prominent Boston architect Guy Lowell, remembered
for his design of the Boston Museum of Fine Arts and the New York
County Courthouse on Foley Square in Manhattan, drew up blueprints
for both houses. At Natirar he was also responsible for the general
estate layout and landscape plan. The Harvard and MIT-educated
architect was assisted by notable New Jersey-born architect Henry
Janeway Hardenbergh who Walter knew of through his iconic hotel
buildings in New York City, Washington, D.C., and Boston.

Kate and Walter were first introduced to Lowell's work through
his design of a prominent new public structure in Bar Harbor called
Building of the Arts. It was a red-tile roofed theater built in the style
of a neo-classical temple. For decades after its completion the theater
was known for featuring world-class entertainment, transforming Bar
Harbor into a summer cultural mecca. Patrons eagerly attended
performances by the Boston Symphony Orchestra and such
luminaries as pianists Jan Paderewski and Joseph Hoffman and master
violinist Fritz Kreisler. One season when all three of the men
presented multiple programs, Kate was ecstatic. To her way of
thinking, this was a "wonderful summer of thrills."[11]

Natirar was the Ladd's primary residence; it was a forty-room,
33,000 square foot Tudor-style mansion. The overall aesthetic of the
mansion was proper and sedate and perhaps reflective of both
Lowell's restrained Boston Brahmin background and Kate's Quaker
upbringing. In keeping with a more reserved aesthetic, Natirar was
constructed of brick with limestone trim. Built in about two years
time, the slate-roofed house featured teak floors, oak paneling,
molded plaster ceilings, and fireplaces in most rooms. The generously

proportioned living room was finished with carved oak and linenfold paneling, and south facing windows provided sweeping views on a clear day. Upstairs, the less-public space where the bedrooms and baths were located, was more simple and austere, spare the lovely mantle pieces found in rooms on either side of the corridor. The third floor, the most Spartan area of the house, contained quarters for servants as well as space for storage. When complete the estate included separate brick staff dwellings, a large greenhouse, which provided flowers for inside the mansion, and a brick coach barn and livery stable, which would one day house automobiles.

Beginning in 1905 and until 1912, when the Natirar mansion was completed, Kate, Walter, and Alice lived in the former Belcher residence. These were Kate's halcyon years and as she fondly recalled,

We moved into Natirar, the old Belcher house in the Spring of 1905. We were a little crowded, but oh, such a happy eight years; practically no illness, and few deaths of our dear ones, so that it seemed as if a new life had come to me, for each year brought more and more physical strength. Miss Lemley and I took a walk each day, and I was able to walk to the station. I did a lot of skating and tobogganing; in fact led a most active life in every direction... those happy days in the old house at Natirar were, in many ways, the best days of my life—really the first time in my life that I had

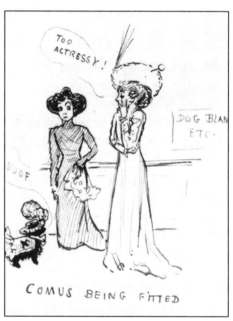

From an original drawing by cartoonist William Ely Hill *(Courtesy of Diane and Craig Conrad)*

known what it was to be really well. How wonderful to awake in the morning without ache or pain, and know I had strength to carry me through the day without straining every nerve and muscle to keep up.[12]

We see that Kate was far from an invalid in those days.

In 1906 Kate found a new source of joy when she and Alice

welcomed a small black Volpino pup, more commonly known in
Britain and America as a Pomeranian, into her home. They named
him Comus.[13] He was a bright-eyed and comical fellow who brought
to mind the dogs that she and Alice had been amused to watch while
touring in Venice, the Volpino having been a fairly common breed of
dog in Italy during the Victorian and Edwardian eras. The so-called
"puffball of dogdom" was favored by both the Italian Queen
Margherita and Queen Victoria.[14] The British Queen had received her
first Pomeranian, "Marco," in Florence in 1888, and she is credited
with popularizing the breed, which was considered to be the height of
fashion by 1906. Affluent Americans (overwhelmingly women) paid
tremendous sums of money for dogs bred in England. It was not
unheard of for a well-bred Pomeranian to cost about $1,200, almost
triple the annual salary of the average New Yorker. After 1910, The
American Pomeranian Club held regular shows at the posh Waldorf
Astoria. These were "exclusive and fashionable" affairs attended by
wealthy women and debutantes.[15]

As might be expected, Comus became a substitute child for Kate.
In an age before dogs were such highly valued family members as
they can be today, Comus was Kate's beloved little boy. At mealtime,
he had a special chair so that he could occupy a place at the table.
This must have seemed highly peculiar to Kate's liveried servants
(whom some guests called "footmen") and outsiders. Weighing no
more than five pounds, Comus posed with Kate for charming
photographs, typically Comus was perched on Kate's shoulder or
snuggled in the crook of her arm. She fussed over him to such an
extent that her "nephew" cartoonist William Ely Hill drew a
humorous cartoon lampooning the little fellow and his mistress. Hill
titled it, "Comus Being Fitted," and the setting is a fashionable shop
where a well-dressed society lady (presumably Kate) wearing an
oversized hat festooned with a gigantic feather and hat pin looks over
a diminutive black Pom. He is outfitted like an over-the-top cavalier
in a ruffled coat and a hat topped with a plume that is as big as he is.
An attractive shop assistant observes the scene with raised eyebrows
as Kate gives Comus the once-over and proclaims that the look is
"Too Actressy!" True to his breed, Comus was a perfect four-legged
companion—intelligent, vivacious, sweet-natured and long-lived.
When he died, Kate mourned his loss as if he had been her child and

she buried Comus in a place of honor close to the front door of her mansion so that she could easily visit his little grave each day.

Chapter 25

AS KATE REVELED IN HER NEWFOUND HEALTH and joy of life at the Belcher farm, she and Alice made preparations for their convalescent home. In 1906, the Ladds purchased a 120-acre parcel of land contiguous to their estate, from Chandler and Mallie Riker. Riker, the founder of a prominent Newark law firm had purchased the one-time Christopher Tiger farm in 1901 for use as a country place. The parcel overlooked the little town of Peapack and it included several outbuildings and a sizable farmhouse which Kate and Alice sought to transform into a comfortable convalescent home. They christened it "Maple Cottage," in homage to the maple trees that stood sentinel in the front yard. Although she did not invoke their names publicly, Kate dedicated her new philanthropic venture to the memory of her parents, Caroline Louise Everit and Josiah Macy Jr.

As they refined their concept of Maple Cottage, Kate and Alice found inspiration in the life and work of Florence Nightingale, the esteemed English nurse and heroine of the Crimean War who subsequently became known as the founder of modern nursing. She believed that no patient should stay longer in a hospital than "absolutely essential" for medical or surgical treatment and asked, "What then should be done with those who are not fit for work-a-day life?" Nightingale opined that every hospital should have a convalescent branch and that every county should have a convalescent home, a place where individuals could rest, receive nourishment, and recuperate in the fresh air. She suggested that convalescents be considered "guests" in an era when patients were frequently called "inmates."[1]

In a black and white photograph Maple Cottage is revealed as it appeared early in its reincarnation as a convalescent home for women. The photographer was local resident Edythe Lane Van Doren. Not more than twenty years old when she purchased her Ascot Number 41 bellows camera, she started her own business snapping local scenes to be printed and sold as postcards.[2] From behind the camera's lens, Van Doren focused on a comfortable white wood-framed structure, newly painted, with a center gable, numerous windows, and a wrap-around porch where guests could rest on rocking chairs and enjoy the bucolic view. Maple Cottage was designed to welcome between fifteen and twenty women at a time in a freshly decorated two-story home. Large windows furnished ample sunlight both upstairs and down. Guests relaxed and enjoyed three nourishing meals daily in a dining room arranged with intimate linen-clothed tables further enhanced by handsome white china inscribed "Maple Cottage" and vases filled with fresh flowers.

Once the site for Maple Cottage was secured and repairs were underway, choosing a competent woman to serve as the home's nursing superintendent was a top priority. Kate had endured the rule of coarse, unqualified matrons at sanitaria in New York and Europe on several occasions and she vehemently opposed hiring such an individual to oversee Maple Cottage. With her background as a graduate nurse, Alice concurred. She championed the selection of a temperate woman with graduate nurse training, a woman who would bring maturity, compassion, and nursing skills to the role of superintendent and share Kate's vision of Maple Cottage as a

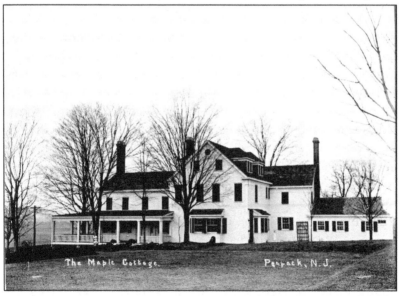

Maple Cottage in winter, circa 1908 by Edythe Lane Van Doren

restorative haven for deserving gentlewomen. The model candidate would oversee the daily operation of the convalescent home, manage staff, and coordinate basic medical services if required.

Two decades had passed since Alice had been a nurse in training. Nevertheless, she retained numerous ties with her alma mater, the "Old Blockley" Hospital in Philadelphia, and hoped that this would be helpful as she searched for an ideal nurse.

In 1884, Blockley had established its nurse training program with the help of Florence Nightingale, whose student, Alice Fisher, was selected to serve as Chief Nurse, thus launching the first American nursing program led by a Nightingale-educated nurse. Alice Lemley's older sister Lily was one of twenty-five women who graduated from the program in 1887.[3] A particularly gifted student, she was awarded the school's prestigious Gold Medal at her fall graduation. It is likely that Lily was Alice's first choice for the job at Maple Cottage. Nonetheless, by the time that the New Jersey convalescent home had become a reality, she was living in Toronto, Canada, where she was comfortably employed as a private nurse companion to Mrs. Minnie Beardmore, a wealthy Canadian matron. Lily had no desire to leave her charmed world of society functions and pleasant summer holidays. After Minnie Beardmore's daughter Lady Constance had married Rear Admiral Sir Charles Kingsmill, Minnie clung to the young woman and treated her like family. She introduced the nurse to her favorite nephew David Livingstone McKeand and would host a large celebration in honor of Lily's late-in-life marriage to him.[4] Once Alice realized that her sister had set her sights on Captain McKeand, she began to look further afield for a nurse supervisor. Ultimately, she and Kate hired Miss H. (Harmony) Estelle Dudley, a fellow graduate of the Blockley class of 1888.

Estelle was one of five children raised in a tight-knit agricultural community west of Syracuse, New York where Dudleys had farmed for generations. Her family placed a high value on education, even for their daughters Estelle and Emma, who would always work to support themselves. Prior to becoming a nurse, Estelle studied to be a teacher at the National Kindergarten Normal School in Washington, D.C. In late 1880, at the age of twenty-eight, she opened a small kindergarten school in Rochester, NewYork in an era when this was an innovative concept. She resided with her aunt and namesake, Harmony Smith

Dudley, and two cousins, Arthur Smith Dudley and Dr. Cynthia Smith, a graduate of the highly regarded Women's Medical College of Pennsylvania. Dr. Smith operated health dispensaries for poor women before her premature death. Her devotion to her profession influenced Arthur to become a doctor and Estelle to leave the field of education and seek a new career in nursing. At age thirty-six she moved to Philadelphia and enrolled in the Blockley nurse training program; Arthur attended medical school at the University of Pennsylvania.

"Stella," as she was known within the family, graduated from the prescribed one-year nursing course in the same class as "Allie" Lemley. Their studies included detailed lectures (presented by male doctors) on topics such as women's nervous disorders and associated surgical procedures including ovariotomy. Students were required to take copious notes which were graded by the lecturer; the notes would serve as helpful guides in practice. For example, in March of 1888 Alice wrote,

> Nervous patients are sometimes seized with night terrors and the nurse should at once reassure her and try to soothe her by holding her hand or by giving ipecac which will generally provoke vomiting and have a soothing effect on Hysteria. If the nurse does not wish to give this, she should rub the arms or put a piece of ice down the patient's back or cold water on head.[5]

The women commenced their careers in Philadelphia, Alice as a private duty nurse and Estelle as the supervisor of the Women's Insane Department at Blockley Hospital. Although Estelle was a prolific writer, no account from her year or so supervising the female insane ward has survived. It appears that she resigned her post in October 1889 and by the early 1890s, had begun to follow private duty nursing, which took her to New York City, the place she called the "big city of lights." Throughout the decade and into the new century, Estelle's work kept her in and around the city. Private duty nursing positions were readily available and provided flexibility for the nurse. Estelle could work when she wanted to and return to the peace of her hometown of Meridian as she wished. In 1898 she built a home for herself on Pearl Street, to have a place to stay when in town. The nurse was always close with her family and throughout much of her tenure in New York City, relatives lived with her.

Estelle's independence and sense of adventure became apparent once she began to travel farther afield from New York. In 1904, she spent a few months with her brother Leland, an artist in delicate health, and his wife Cora in Southern Pines, North Carolina. Rather than lull around on holiday, she intended to offer "lessons in scientific and correct breathing" at her temporary home at Piney View Cottage.[6] Perhaps these lessons were meant to advance the health of people like her brother who sought out the dry and mild winter climate and pine scented fresh air of Southern Pines as an antidote to respiratory problems. By the winter of 1906, her thirst for adventure had deepened and led her to Los Angeles where she worked for a Dr. Juliette. Even though she missed her family a great deal, the nurse was having the time of her life in California. She wrote letters home regularly and extolled her numerous off-duty activities telling her niece Jeanie that she was "getting on famously with French," had resumed the study of German, belonged to an Emerson class and a Whist club, and was "doing considerable writing all the time." Intrigue associated with a speculative deal added an entirely new kind of excitement to her life: One of her employer's "intimate friends" had invented a marine engineering device that was expected to change the way the nation built bridges, forts, lighthouses, and torpedo stations and bring untold riches to investors. Since Dr. Juliette was on the project's board of directors, Estelle was privy to "all the inside news that the general public knows nothing about." It appears that she invested some of her savings in the project because she wrote that it would not be bad if she could use "six figures to express my fortune." "Aunt Stella" told her niece that she "would not leave here now for anything—it's getting too exciting and I want to watch the game out."[7]

Nevertheless, a year later Estelle abruptly returned to the east. Most of her family continued to live in upstate New York; her cousin Arthur was now practicing medicine in New Brunswick, New Jersey. Her brother was living by the Jersey Shore at Long Branch. No one discussed what had occurred to terminate her exciting interlude in the City of Angels, but the timing of her homecoming turned out to be providential: Alice approached Estelle with an offer to manage the new convalescent home in New Jersey.

After Kate met with Miss Dudley, she felt convinced about the nurse's suitability for the job. Estelle was a mature woman with well-honed nursing skills, a deep religious faith, and a good sense of humor. Kate also appreciated her eclectic background and interests. In need of an income, Estelle eagerly accepted the position as Maple Cottage's first nurse superintendent. Given that the cottage operated seasonally, from May 1 until October 1, she was free to indulge in other activities during the off-season. Estelle used her annual six months off to enjoy far-flung travel. In her hometown she became highly regarded as an international globetrotter whose thrilling travel stories were published regularly in the local newspaper, the *Cato Citizen*.

Although Maple Cottage was not intended to serve local women, by its second year of operation area residents were well-aware of its existence. The *Bernardsville News* alerted readers to the presence of the "Convalescents' Home on the old Riker place, now part of the Walter G. Ladd estate." It was reported that "a nice class only, of city women to whom everything, including transportation, is absolutely free" were given a two-week stay "in this delightful retreat on the hill overlooking Peapack." It was explained that Maple Cottage was Mrs. Ladd's way of showing her gratitude for recovering her health after a long period of invalidism. The news article further commented that Miss H. Estelle Dudley was "the efficient and kindly superintendent of this unique and helpful institution, which fitly represents Christianity in action."[8]

Not long thereafter, glowing words about Maple Cottage spread far beyond New York and New Jersey when *The American Journal of Nursing* published a letter to the editor titled *An Unusual Opportunity For Nurses In Need Of Rest*. Coincidentally, the author was a graduate of the New York Hospital's nurse training program, the hospital where Kate's grandfather had been involved for decades and where Kate was first exposed to the needs of the infirm.

Dear Editor: I am at present enjoying the hospitality of a beautiful place, "Maple Cottage," provided by Mrs. Walter G. Ladd, where she invites educated self-supporting women in need of rest and recuperation to visit as her guests, without money and price.

Mrs. Ladd has herself been a great sufferer from ill health and been ministered to by graduate nurses. She has thought much about the needs of her suffering fellow women and out of her boundless sympathy and unlimited means supports this delightful abode, where women may come for the needed rest and care to restore them to health that they may resume the duties of their vocations by which they make themselves independent.

Mrs. Ladd does not offer this as a charity, though, there is no pay accepted. And from New York return tickets are supplied. It is just "her way" of doing good, and she earnestly wishes nurses, teachers, artists, and all self-supporting women of education and refinement who may be benefited by a stay at Maple Cottage, to accept her most cordial invitation.

Miss Dudley, a graduate nurse, looks after the guests in a most capable and delightful manner, making everyone feel at home and most welcome.

All communications should be addressed to Miss H. Estelle Dudley, Superintendent, Maple Cottage, Peapack, N.J.

Matilda Agnes Frederick, R.N.[9]

Kate later recalled the day when she and Alice received their first guests at Maple Cottage as "the happiest day of my life." She noted that for years she spent a great deal of time over at the cottage but credited her superintendent Estelle Dudley's "beautiful spirit and good management" for making Maple Cottage such a success.[10]

While Estelle was praised for her kindness and beautiful spirit, her early life in an out-of-the-way farming community led her to become a thrifty and practical woman and her successful management of the convalescent home was largely due to her ability to run a tight and orderly ship. One concrete expression of Estelle's firm management was the set of ten concise guidelines that she established for cottage guests. A typed memo on official Maple Cottage letterhead decreed that no woman suffering from a mental disease or chronic illness such as consumption, epilepsy, or cancer would be admitted to the Home. Neither women under the age of seventeen nor elderly women were eligible for a stay at Maple Cottage; all guests were expected to be ambulatory and able to "wait upon themselves." Furthermore, if routine medical treatment was required, house rules stipulated that it would be furnished by a doctor connected with the cottage. In the event a guest became more seriously ill during a stay, the place of treatment would be determined at the discretion of the superintendent who made it known that all "Persons admitted must conform to such house rules and other rules and regulations as may be from time to time promulgated."[11]

Guests at Maple Cottage appreciated that they were well-nourished both physically and spiritually. As superintendent, Estelle was responsible for planning the healthful meals served each day. Never one to put butter upon bacon, she maintained a large ledger book filled with simple recipes (many of these had been given to her by friends and relatives in Meridian) and household advice aimed at providing the best in convalescent fare without breaking the bank. A glimpse at her Maple Cottage ledger book reveals scores of recipes written in Estelle's neat hand. They cover every manner of food—fish, meat, soups, eggs, vegetables, breads, biscuits, muffins, pies and cakes, ice cream and sherbets. Directions for canning and preserving summer's bounty were readily available. Many recipes including Dr. Bradford's Laxative Bread, Cynthia Smith's rice pudding, and "Soft-boiled eggs Mrs. Rover's way" seem to fit the bill for convalescent fare in that era—others, such as Irish Stew, Mexican frijoles, onions on toast and sweet pickled cantaloupe, far less so. "Mrs. Ladd's Cook's Ginger Cake" and other desserts prepared with ginger, molasses and graham flour figured prominently in Estelle's expansive cookery collection. Her ledger also provided household hints ranging from effective methods of stain removal to dandruff cures, antidotes for poison ivy, and "death to cockroaches"—step-by-step directions for the eradication of the unpleasant creature were furnished courtesy of one of the numerous popular ladies magazines of the era.

To a great extent, Kate was responsible for providing her guests with a healthy measure of spiritual nourishment. She ensured that the atmosphere at the Cottage was always gracious and accommodating; the many small luxuries provided for guests throughout the years were uniformly her doing. A bookworm since her student days with Julia Nott, Kate personally found literature to be an important source of uplift. She sought to share her love of reading with her Maple Cottage guests by establishing a library on the grounds of the convalescent home. The Maple Cottage Library, housed in a one and one half story building with a slope-roofed front porch, became one of her pet projects. Kate eagerly selected a diverse mix of books and periodicals for the enjoyment of her guests and stocked the shelves with classics as well as the works of authors she knew personally including the fictional novels of Dr. S. Weir Mitchell and the poetry of Angela Morgan, who was considered to be a leader in the ranks of the younger American poets. She dedicated *Utterance and Other Poems* to Kate, her good friend Emily Vanderbilt Hammond, and Mrs. Andrew Carnegie—the women were the author's most significant patrons. One season, Miss Morgan visited Kate at Natirar and presented an "entertainment" to the guests at Maple Cottage.[12] For those women who were less inclined to linger on the porch with a serious book, there were always magazines to peruse: *The Cosmopolitan* (the precursor to the modern fashion magazine, originally a family and literary magazine), *The Ladies' World, Ladies' Home Journal, The Century Illustrated Monthly Magazine,* and Estelle Dudley's favorite periodical, the *National Geographic Magazine,* were devoured by guests along with millions of Americans in the early twentieth century.

In addition to furnishing the women of Maple Cottage with a convenient place to borrow a wide range of reading material, Kate compiled and published two unique and charming volumes of inspirational prose, *Autumn Leaves From Maple Cottage* and *Spring Blossoms From Maple Cottage*. These little-known books, precursors to the proliferation of inspirational literature available in the twenty-first century, are treasures. They were Kate's gift to her guests, intended to add further comfort and support during their stay in Peapack as well as when they returned to their work-a-day lives.

Kate introduced each book with a brief foreword.

Autumn Leaves From Maple Cottage,

As one gathers autumn leaves, some on their own branch, some brought together by friendly winds, so have thoughts and visions and some sayings of others been gathered together on these pages for the comfort of those who might be in real need of them. They have been lived and have helped and now may they help others and link themselves pleasantly to the memory of the days spent at Maple Cottage.

And in *Spring Blossoms From Maple Cottage* she wrote,

Hope renewed, courage reborn, beauty unfolding anew its buds of life—such has seemed to me the meaning of Spring. After the silence of snow and the waiting wondering of winter sleep, branch and bird speak up again in their way of greeting the coming Spring. With balm and breeze another feast of color and song and

love prepares the glory of the Spirit of Life. To believe, to begin
again to hold fast to courage and purpose is the message with
which these Spring-blossoms from Maple Cottage may greet its
weary guests and comfort their parting.[13]

Thirty years after Kate and Alice opened the doors of their
convalescent home to working women in need of respite, guests
continued to find solace and joy in their two-week stay in Peapack, as
evidenced by the words of one guest. They were written on the back
of a picture postcard of Maple Cottage and sent to a friend who lived
on West Twelfth Street in New York City,

> The days have slipped away to the cry of the crow, in the
> meadow, the hum of insect life in the gardens and the glorious
> sunshine over all. These last two mornings I heard the strong
> crowing of a cock from the farm yard up the road, who has
> undoubtedly been attending to business all the while I slept—and
> how I have rested! My comfortable cot bed is at an angle of two
> large windows from which I get a view of the lawn and the road
> passing. It has been a joy to have this glorious change after several
> years of Manhattan brick, cement, and dirty atmosphere plus noise.
> Long walks and fresh air, with rolling hills of many autumn colors,
> refresh mind and spirit, I hope to find you rested, well and ready
> for the coming winter.

My best wishes,
Josephine Isadore Burroughs.[14]

It is estimated that through the caring efforts of Kate Macy Ladd,
Alice Lemley, Estelle Dudley and staff, as well as through Kate's
enduring generosity, more than 4,000 women were able to rest and
recuperate on the Natirar estate at the compassionate haven known as
Maple Cottage.

Chapter 26

KATE'S BLESSINGS MULTIPLIED THROUGHOUT her early golden years at Natirar. As Maple Cottage flourished so did her health, community involvement, and enjoyment of life. Although faint traces of their footsteps exist in various places such as in the beautiful stained glass windows at St. Bernards Church in Bernardsville, the Ladds are virtually unknown to residents of Somerset County and Bar Harbor today. This may be in part because Kate made a career of philanthropy without fanfare, just as her mother had done before her. A little known but important Macy family account of Carrie's beneficence tells how in the early 1890s, the board of the original New York College for the Training of Teachers sought a source of funds to expand school facilities. It was probably Kate's brother (who was interested in manual arts education) who brought the proposed project to his mother's attention. To the great surprise of the board of trustees, in February 1893 two gentlemen representing Carrie Macy offered the sum of $200,000 to "erect and equip" a building as a memorial to her husband. The men stipulated that the donation remain anonymous until such time as "the lady" wished to make it known.[1] Kate's mother's largesse resulted in Macy Hall, a five-story secular Gothic building which became the home to a preeminent teacher training school and is today affiliated with Columbia University.[2] While Kate's brother is well-remembered for his fourteen years as chairman of the board of trustees of Teachers College and for being awarded an honorary Doctor of Laws degree from Columbia, Carrie Macy's role in funding the building is virtually unknown.

Once they had become homeowners the Ladds regularly moved about from one residence to another. Between October and June they were based in New Jersey, at Natirar, or in New York City where they leased apartments in luxury hotels such as the Plaza and the St. Regis. For several years the Ladds had gone south for a few months after spending Christmas at Natirar to such renowned winter playgrounds for the rich as Jekyll Island and Augusta, Georgia; Pinehurst, North Carolina; and Palm Beach, Florida. By 1912 Kate was feeling so good that she rebelled against spending her winters away from home. She preferred to remain up north so that she could make weekly trips to the city to enjoy time with friends, see family, and attend performances at the cultural venues she had loved since her youth. She frequented performances at the old Metropolitan Opera House on Thirty-Ninth Street where the Ladds always had a box for the season; at one point, they rented parterre box fourteen, which was shared with the well-known financier, philanthropist, and chairman of the Met, Otto H. Kahn.[3] Kate also attended the symphony and theater (which she had renounced as a young woman, in part to please her grandmother), took classes in literature exploring the mysteries of the ancient *Bagavad Gita,* and participated in her Visiting Nurse and social workers' meetings, often accompanied by Alice.

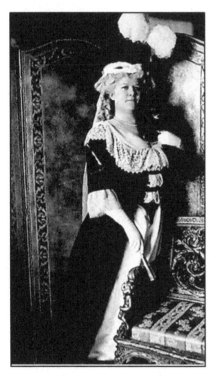

Kate, age 46 (*Courtesy of Diane and Craig Conrad*)

From 1905 until early 1917, she enjoyed a full and meaningful life as she reviewed in her Line-A-Day Diary:

Edytha Macy (sic. Everit's youngest child) is with us, and I read aloud to her this morning. At   one, Walter and I went to the Clarence Blair Mitchell's to lunch; forty-two there. Edytha came for us after lunch and we motored to New York. She and I went to see Chester and Amy Aldrich, also called on Agnes. I then took her home; had massage, and went in the evening to the opera with Walter to hear Manon Lescaut.

Kate emphasized that all her days were like this, "and some even fuller." [4] Undoubtedly, she was delighted to be healthy and on-the-go.

During the summer months Alice spent most of her time in Maine at Eegonos, where her bedroom adjoined Kate's. Nonetheless, the Ladds recognized that she would benefit from having a place to call her own, a spot to comfortably entertain her sisters, nieces and nephews, and friends. Kate and Walter built and attractively furnished a comfortable waterfront cottage for her in a bungalow community called Shady Nook in Trent, Maine. Kate was Alice's first guest. She gave her a green leather-bound guest book as a housewarming gift. In it she wrote, "Glorious day sunshine within and without. To all those who may dwell therein from generation to generation may it be a house of God, a gate of heaven." The book records the names and comments of Alice's visitors. In addition to her Pennsylvania kin and friends and the McKeands from Ottawa, the Ladds and many of Kate's friends and relatives were among Alice's regular visitors.[5] It would have warmed Kate's heart to know that the bungalow remained in Alice's family for generations and that throughout this time large

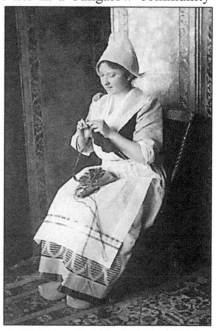

Alice Lemley, age 39 *(Courtesy of Diane and Craig Conrad)*

framed photographs of Kate, in fancy dress, and Alice dressed like a Dutch girl, hung side-by-side in the bungalow's living room. Kate's photograph is especially charming. She wears an eighteenth century ruffled gown and an elaborate hat which cover a white wig; ringlets skim her shoulders. Kate is standing and holds Comus securely on her left shoulder with a gloved hand. She is forty-six years old and her full face and peaceful gaze suggest that she is in the absolute pink of health.

Forever devoted to her siblings, Kate especially enjoyed entertaining their children. During the summer of 1913 she hosted

Everit's younger son Noel and daughter Edytha at Eegonos; they were
kept busy from morning until night. Their mother Edith wrote to her
son from her Catskill Mountain home Hathaway,

> What a glorious time Aunt Kate is giving you and Edytha.
> Imagine having a yachting party arranged for the infants, I never
> heard of anything so thrilling. Give my best to Aunt Kate and tell
> her I hope she did not find the experience exhausting- we know
> how much   parties take out of the hosts sometimes and it seems to
> me that Aunt Kate has been entertaining pretty continuously on
> *Walucia.*

Walucia was a luxury steam yacht, and for the Macy children,
ages twelve and nine, the opportunity to spend days cruising the
waters around Mt. Desert Island was like something from a dream.
The youngsters were also treated to visits at Alice's new bungalow
where they could skip stones at the water's edge and warm their toes
in the sand. They were among the first to sign the green guestbook:
Noel wrote "SWELL!!!!" in bold letters in the column reserved for
"remarks."

By this time Kate's hellish summer at Elsinore was completely
behind her. She had become an enthusiastic member of the Mt. Desert
Island summer colony and fully embraced her husband's love of the
popular pastime of yachting. She found days on the water to be
relaxing and comfortable and loved entertaining as they sailed. The
Ladds leased a yacht each season until they purchased what Kate
called "our own beautiful *Wenonah.*" The craft, which was
constructed in Neponset, Massachusetts by the firm of George Lawley
and Sons, was delivered to Eegonos in August 1915. According to
Kate, a more perfect vessel never sailed the waters; she thrilled to see
the 164-foot, steel-hulled steam yacht anchored off Eegonos.[6] The
Ladds were as smitten with the *Wenonah* as a middle-aged couple
might have been with a long-awaited grandchild. Her virtues were
hailed in the *Boston Daily Globe.* The newspaper reported that the
Wenonah was "a handsome addition to the New York Yacht Club
fleet."[7]

> Beginning well aft toward the stern, below deck is a large
> double stateroom, the four single staterooms and two bathrooms
> and the owner's double stateroom, taking the full width of the
> vessel, with a private bathroom forward of these...The owner's
> and guest quarters are finished in white with mahogany trim.[8]

The Ladds' new acquisition was truly exceptional. The *Wenonah's* captain and engineer had private staterooms; the crew had their own quarters as well as a mess room. The Ladds and their guests enjoyed the yacht's large saloon and dining room. A favorite pastime was the luncheon cruise where Kate sometimes entertained female friends including such notable women as Virginia Gildersleeve, Dean of Barnard College, Lillian Wald, founder of the Visiting Nurse Association, and Martha McChesney Berry who established the Berry School in the Blue Ridge Mountains in Georgia. Sadly, Kate and Walter's enjoyment of the *Wenonah* was short-lived. The U.S. government confiscated her for the war effort in June 1917. During World War I, the *U.S.S. Wenonah* escorted convoys between Gibraltar and Bizerte, Tunisia, countering combat between Gibraltar and Genoa, Italy in 1918. Although she missed the yacht, Kate graciously acknowledged that "She did good work, so we must not murmur."[9]

The Ladds spent part of the summer of 1915 at home. According to the local Peapack newspaper, it was not until the third week in July that they traveled up to Bar Harbor, conveying "forty trunks and a carload of horses."[10] Kate had her first swimming lesson that summer and said that she had entertained "continual house guests from May to October; dinner parties, musicals, etc."[11]

With her newfound energy Kate became involved in a variety of activities at her summer home. She particularly enjoyed hosting dinner parties followed by musicales in her spacious music room overlooking Frenchman's Bay. Well-loved performers of the day, such as the popular tenor George Harris and the Schroeder Trio, delighted her guests. Her love of music extended to her enjoyment of the programs at Building of Arts where she regularly engaged a box and witnessed performances by the European-born divas, soprano Alma Gluck and mezzo-soprano Margarete Matzenauer. Each summer she was a patroness of the annual Hampton Institute Folk Concerts. Hampton was dedicated to the education African American and Native American boys and under the direction of Dr. R. Nathaniel Dett, the school became internationally known for its acclaimed Choir and Quartet. Dr. Dett and his students made an annual appearance in Bar Harbor which introduced the public to Hampton and its mission; the tours became a lucrative method of fundraising. Kate was so taken by the students that she became a dedicated financial supporter. And Hampton Institute (as it was called from 1930-1984 before the school was renamed Hampton University) would eventually become a major beneficiary of the Ladds' largesse. Kate's interests in literature and the natural world also found expression in Bar Harbor. She helped to advance the early writing career of the up-and-coming poet Angela Morgan, who spent ten days at Eegonos during which time Kate introduced her to other wealthy society women. She also sponsored a regular series of nature lectures presented by "Miss Marshall" in her home. Throughout this period she participated in charity work to benefit the Young Women's Christian Association with her dear friend Alice Vanderbilt Morris, a brilliant linguist who founded the International Auxiliary Language Association in 1924. All the while, entertaining family members and New York friends at her summer refuge continued to be a joyful priority.

While in residence at Natirar, the Ladds hosted several sizable events. They "gave a large dance and over one hundred people came," as Kate recalled. "We seated one hundred and ten people at supper in our large living-room, and some of the young people on the terrace."[12] On another occasion, with every bedroom occupied by visitors, Kate was making final preparations for a concert for over a hundred guests when Walter took a fall from his horse that left him seriously injured. Kate wanted to cancel the gathering but Walter would hear nothing of it, saying that if the event was cancelled, he would get out of bed against doctor's orders. As a result, Kate received their guests alone and the concert proceeded as planned.[13]

Walter convalesced slowly, and although Kate was attentive to his needs she continued to enjoy herself. She tried tobogganing for the first time (at age fifty-two) and crowed about doing a lot of skating. She also relished weekly visits to her apartment in the city. When Walter recovered they attended a spectacular dinner dance for more than 200 guests at the Fifth Avenue residence of the young widow Mrs. John J. Astor. Gold dinner service and pink flowers enlivened the dining room and, according to one newspaper account, an additional 150 guests arrived for dancing and a supper in the picture gallery at 1 a.m. In her memoir Kate described the Astor party as "one of the largest private dinners ever given in New York."[14] The Ladds were acquainted with Mrs. Astor through Bar Harbor friends as well as Macy family connections: Madeline Force Astor would give up her inherited fortune to marry William K. Dick later that year. Dick's sister Julia was married to William Kingsland Macy, the youngest son of Kate's favorite cousin George.

During these busy years she was always eager to try new things. Kate did some "motoring" for the first time—the advent of the automobile introduced a new era of travel for the affluent and Kate was not to be left out. She and Alice took an extensive trip by chauffeured automobile. They motored to Rochester, New York, to visit Macy cousins Bunnie and Lillie, and went on to Niagara Falls to meet Alice's sister Lily. The women traveled 1,300 miles by car and Kate said that she enjoyed every moment although she acknowledged having missed the company of Walter who "hated to motor."[15] Regarding auto travel, Kate was far more like her brother Everit. He was a great auto enthusiast and one of nine founding directors of the American Automobile Club—by 1906 he and his wife Edith were known to travel by chauffeured automobile whenever possible and perhaps this rubbed off on Kate. Rather than take the train, Kate and Alice motored to Philadelphia for the sad occasion of the funeral of their friend S. W. Mitchell. Dr. Mitchell's funeral was held at St. Stephen's Episcopal Church, which had been built upon the original site of Benjamin Franklin's legendary eighteenth century electrical experiments. Augustus Saint-Gauden's solemn marble sculpture "The Angel of Purity," which had been commissioned by the Mitchells years before in remembrance of their daughter Maria, was in full view, lending further poignancy to an occasion that would all too soon be repeated. Mrs. Maria Mitchell died nine days after her famous husband. Kate commented that the church was crowded with young and old, rich and poor, all intent upon honoring Dr. Mitchell remarking, "I have never seen such crowds, extending far into the middle of the street."[16] Kate's devotion toward the Mitchell family continued long after the deaths of the doctor and his wife. Acknowledging that for many years he had been the guiding spirit behind the original Orthopedic Hospital and Infirmary for Nervous Disease in Philadelphia, the Ladds, "his long-time and deeply devoted friends," made a "magnificent gift" in his memory, donating a well-equipped outpatient department building to the hospital where he worked throughout his storied career.[17]

By the time she offered funds for the hospital addition, meant to provide a lasting memorial for Dr. Mitchell, Kate was fully engaged with organizations that supported initiatives aimed at improving health closer to home. In the early years of the twentieth century, possibly through the influence of her social reform-minded sister-in-law Edith Carpenter Macy, Kate was drawn to support the work of public nursing advocate Lillian Wald who had been ministering among the poor of New York City since 1893. Miss Wald was not a typical nurse. Unlike Alice and Estelle, women who came from small towns and families with little money to spare for luxuries, Wald was raised in a comfortable and refined atmosphere. Her father was a successful businessman and provided his daughter with the advantage of a fine education. She had attended an English-French boarding school in Rochester, New York, and graduated from the New York Hospital Training School for Nurses (an affiliate of the New York Hospital where Kate's Grandfather served for many years) with an eye to train further for a career in medicine. She attended classes at the Women's Medical College of the New York Infirmary founded by Drs. Elizabeth and Emily Blackwell. However, while working with impoverished immigrants on the crowded Lower East Side of New York City she had a change of heart, giving up her medical studies to minister to the poor as a full-time community health nurse. At the request of Jacob Schiff, the wealthy Jewish financier and philanthropist, Wald provided instruction on home nursing and hygiene for neighborhood women at a building he furnished on Henry Street. The classes were successful and the curriculum expanded to include instruction in English, sewing, and cooking. Cultural programs followed along with daycare and playground facilities for children. Initially known as "The Nurses' Settlement," Miss Wald's efforts spawned what became known as the Henry Street Settlement and the Visiting Nurse Service of New York City. By 1913, Wald was well-known nationwide. She managed a staff of 92 nurses, dedicated to serving the health and welfare of those in need. Remarkably in 1933, the year of her retirement, her staff numbered 265 nurses; they served some 100,000 patients city-wide.

Wald's cadre of nurses was supported by an association largely comprised of wealthy and charitable individuals such as Kate and Edith who became her personal friends. The sisters-in-law attended regular meetings of the Visiting Nurse Association in New York. The association supported all aspects of the nurses' work including overseeing the funding of their salaries and making community programs possible.[18] Edith's individual efforts were widely praised; for years she and her husband sent fresh milk from their farm in Westchester County to nourish hundreds of babies at the Henry Street Settlement. Ensuring the availability of wholesome milk for children was an issue that Kate would also champion in New Jersey where she naturally gravitated toward participation with the Somerset Hills Visiting Nurse Association based near her home at Natirar.

In 1903, the Somerset Hills had a fleeting taste of what public health nursing could provide when the St. Bernard's Episcopal Church in Bernardsville hired a parish nurse to minister to the sick and poor. Despite her efforts, it quickly became apparent that her services were not being fully utilized because the neediest members of the community perceived her to be a messenger of the Episcopal Church. In recognition of this situation, a group of public-minded women formed a committee to examine the issue; they determined the need to employ a nonsectarian nurse. In 1906, the Visiting Nurse Association of Bernardsville was born; a short time later the group expanded and became known as the Visiting Nurse Association of Somerset Hills. The following year Kate was listed as a "subscriber" (supporter) of the organization. She remained an active member throughout her life and is remembered for her service on the board of trustees and for her service on the executive and nursing committees.[19]

Kate knew that the work of her local branch of the Visiting Nurse Association was enormously important. Although the Somerset Hills was known to be an elite enclave, the vicinity was also home to a sizable population of immigrant families, those individuals whose toil made it possible to maintain the area's large estates and the affluent residents' luxurious lifestyles. The Ladds were typical members of their colony. They relied upon their employees—housemaids, laundresses, and waiters—to ensure that the mansion ran like clockwork. Walter was known to be so particular about the maintenance of his property that he hired large crews of men to handpick weeds from the great lawn and regularly rake the carriage paths so that his 1,000 acres remained in pristine condition.

However, in the shadow of this opulence, many of the great estates' employees struggled to take care of their families. The local Visiting Nurse Association (or the V.N.A.) saw the need for healthcare services and stepped in to fill the void. Their efforts made a tremendous difference in the well-being of the community particularly once they provided home health visits. The nurses expanded their services to offer home based hygiene education. This initiative was so well-received and deemed so important that it spilled over into the public schools where the association helped to coordinate classroom instruction: Students learned the basics of good nutrition, the correct way to blow the nose, and the importance of using toothpaste. The nurses focused on the issue of dental hygiene and poor vision. Defective teeth were a widespread problem; in 1915, ninety-nine percent of students in Peapack-Gladstone were reported to have bad teeth while many also had vision problems that had never been addressed. To combat these issues the Visiting Nurse Association established dental and vision screenings at school and coordinated the services of dentists and oculists when necessary. Kate's Nurse Committee report for this period stated:

> Sickness alleviated and made easier to bear by trained nursing care, hygiene taught by example, lectures and friendly talks, school children examined, and parents advised while instruction and prevention have been the watchwords of our work.[20]

It is no wonder that participation in the Visiting Nurse Association of Somerset Hills became one of Kate's passions. Meeting minutes and annual reports illuminate the active role she played in the organization. For example, minutes recorded on December 2, 1915, state that "Mr. and Mrs. Ladd have purchased a house in Peapack which they have very generously loaned to the sub-committee (sic Raritan-River) for a year." The Ladds further provided funds to cover a nurse's salary and a car with chauffeur to safely escort her on house calls.[21] Also noted was Kate's invitation to host the next meeting at Natirar, rather than have the group continue to convene at the drafty firehouse on Main Street. Members were instructed to "bring sewing bags to next meeting which will be at Mrs. Ladd's house."[22]

January 6, 1916: If we could quietly slip into Kate's spacious drawing room and settled into a chair by the roaring fireplace, we would join members of the Raritan-River branch of the Visiting Nurse Association. Despite the cold weather, forty-seven well-dressed women had gathered for their monthly meeting. Needle and thread in hand, they stitched away while the business of the day was conducted. Alice was in attendance—her precise needlework admired by all. In contrast to the coarse shirts and shifts that she and Kate once made for the "hungry-eyed" people they encountered along the banks of the Nile, Alice's tiny stitches created soft and delicate items—diapers, slips, caps, and scarves—for the baby layettes that a visiting nurse would deliver to a new mother. While everyone knitted or sewed Kate expressed concern about impure milk, an issue that had been on her mind for some time. She was well-aware of her sister-in-law's efforts to provide wholesome milk to children in New York City and knew that milk quality was a problem in the Somerset Hills as well. In Bernard's Township a baby became "desperately ill" from tainted milk. Kate was alarmed to learn that among forty-four local milk dealers most "were without any idea of sanitation or cleanliness"[23] Kate made a motion from the floor to request that the association contact local boards of health to solicit the appointment of a milk inspector. Her motion was carried and as a result, milk inspections got underway.

We can see that Kate thrived as a board member of the Somerset Hills Visiting Nurse Association. In all likelihood her involvement with Lillian Wald and the Henry Street Settlement provided a strong foundation for her understanding of community health issues.

One month later, despite "disagreeable weather" a contingent of thirty-nine association members convened once again to knit, sew, and discuss organizational business at Natirar. Once again the issue of sanitary milk was on the agenda; "Mrs. Fritz" was appointed to accompany the milk inspectors on their rounds. The women's efforts were enhanced when a local physician agreed to organize a symposium on the subject of pure milk to be held at the Bernards auditorium.

Kate's devotion to the V.N.A. was unwavering. She purchased and organized supplies for the Visiting Nurse Home even though she was suffering from what her doctor called appendix trouble, and her physical discomfort did not stop her from planning a special event for the organization. She invited her friend Lillian Wald to come to

Natirar to speak on the topic of "Visiting Nursing." Miss Wald was a
heroine to women nationwide; her appearance in Peapack was highly
memorable. Seventy association members and guests were on hand
for Miss Wald's "interesting and instructive address."[24] As Kate
recalled, "After her talk we served tea. Miss Wald spent the night here
and we gave a dinner for her that evening. It was a great privilege to
have her in our home and I have always felt a warm friendship for
her."[25] Earlier in the day during the business portion of the meeting a
letter from Walter Ladd was read to the group. He and Kate offered to
donate the Peapack house to the association for the use of the nurses.
The Ladds' generous offer was approved by the executive committee
with "grateful appreciation."[26]

    The Nurses' Home in Peapack bought and equipped by Mr.
and Mrs. Walter G. Ladd fills a long felt want of an adequate home
for the nurse. One must see the home to fully appreciate its charm
and the perfection of arrangement and detail in the operating room.

    Here also Dr. Keim has operated at clinics for adenoids and
tonsils."[27]

Chapter 27

EVEN AS HER FOCUS on the local Visiting Nurse Association grew, Kate remained open to the possibility of taking on additional philanthropic efforts: It was a train trip south by private railroad car that opened the door to another enduring charitable venture. Her brother Everit was able to skillfully motivate her to take action on behalf of those in need; he suggested that Kate investigate the work being done to uplift poor rural youth at the Berry School in Rome, Georgia. He probably made the arrangements for Kate's visit and introduced her to Berry's founder, Martha McChesney Berry. Everit was also an early promoter of Hampton Institute and Tuskegee Normal and Industrial Institute (whose first principal was Booker T. Washington, a former Hampton teacher), and he induced the Ladds to financially support those institutions as well.

Like Kate and her brother, Martha Berry was moved by the plight of those in need. She dedicated her life to improving the lives of impoverished children through education. Miss Berry grew up outside of Rome, Georgia, located about seventy-five miles northwest of Atlanta; her parents were considered members of the landed gentry. Berry's first attempt to educate local children began modestly through the establishment of Sunday schools. These programs evolved into day schools which first served boys and by 1909 girls as well. Known as the Berry School and directed by its founder, the school's early curriculum emphasized practical instruction that would prove useful when students returned to their rural communities. While the boys studied agriculture and mechanics, the girls studied home economics, dairying, and gardening. In addition, all students studied the Bible and basic academic subjects and they were expected to perform work on campus, a requirement that was in force until the early 1960s. Students worked in the dining hall, the laundry, the campus dairy, on construction projects, and in workshops where they learned such traditional skills as weaving and food preservation, creating items to sell to profit the school. In many cases tuition credit was earned through campus labor.

In her memoir Kate wrote, "On March 14, 1915, we had a very interesting and inspiring experience. Walter took a private car, and we invited Mr. and Mrs. Francis Riggs, Augusta Hope, and Miss Lemley to go down to Berry School for a few days."[1] Kate failed to mention that little Comus was in tow. In the minds of the Berry students, who enjoyed his comical antics, he would be as unforgettable a member of the Ladds' traveling party as Mr. Riggs who stood six feet, seven inches tall in his stocking feet.

Whereas Comus provided entertainment, (as when he hid beneath Kate's cape during chapel services, only to jump out barking and offering a tiny paw to the boys and girls who applauded and howled with laughter at this unexpected break in decorum), Francis Riggs's visit had a serious underlying purpose. Riggs, a graduate of Groton and Harvard, and his wife, Valerie Burckhardt Hadden, hailed from prominent moneyed families. They were ardent pacifists and idealists who believed that the eradication of poverty and ignorance could end all future war. They came to Berry to see firsthand what Martha Berry was doing to educate and uplift poor boys and girls. The Riggses were so inspired by what they had observed that they opened the Riggs School in Lakeville, Connecticut, the following year. Over time their endeavor evolved from a small agricultural program for boys into the Indian Mountain School, today an institution providing education for boys and girls from pre-kindergarten through ninth grade in its original location in Connecticut.

Martha Berry, Kate, and Mr. and Mrs. Riggs were united in the belief that all children deserved a relevant education regardless of class. Miss Berry, who never married, considered her students and faculty members to be her family; she utilized every grain of her being to make Berry a vibrant community and a school that moved forward with the times. To do so she depended upon the support of like-minded men and women with means. She reminisced that upon meeting Kate for the first time, "Mrs. Ladd, with Comus under her arm, was like a ray of sunshine, going from one end of campus to the other and soon won the hearts and minds of all the boys and girls and the faculty of the Berry Schools."[2] Kate's popularity may have been enhanced by the simple gifts she brought to campus. During a travel layover in Atlanta, she ordered a box of chocolates for every student from Nunallys, a well-known candy store—she was not prepared for the students' outpouring of appreciation. A young boy told her in his entire life no one had ever given him such a special gift; other students vowed to share their precious confections with younger siblings back home. The children's gratitude touched Kate to such a great extent that she made it a practice to order a box of candy for every Berry student each year at Christmastime. In early December she would send a telegram to Martha Berry, "Please telegraph how many pupils are at Berry as I must give Christmas order."[3] Christmas candy from Mrs. Ladd was a happy holiday tradition for years. Kate's heartwarming experience with the spirited young people at Berry led her to describe her visit to Berry as one of the most thrilling experiences of her life.[4] Alice was similarly inspired by the school and its students. Basking in the afterglow of the visit to Berry, she sent a note to Martha Berry.

> It would be impossible for me to tell you on paper how much enjoyment and inspiration I received during our little visit with you at the school. It was all so perfect that my store-house of pleasant memories is overflowing and it is so delightful to picture it all so vividly, and to see you doing your wonderful work among the pupils. Thank you so many times for all you did to give us so much pleasure and please thank all of our friends too, the faculty and the students, for their kindness.[5]

As Kate later recalled, "Miss Lemley, my dear companion, was so impressed she worked every minute of her spare time and sold the things she made to endow a day at Berry."[6] Endowing a day at Berry was a serious financial commitment: Alice pledged a donation of $1,250 to the school endowment fund, the interest on which would "perpetually help and bless" some boy or girl in need.[7] Her sincerity was widely felt. A school publication, *Southern Highlander,* made Alice's wishes known, "Miss Lemley expressed a desire to have a share in Berry herself saying she had little money but that she would use her 'magic needle' to make lovely things to sell to Mrs. Ladd's friends, and send the money down to Berry.[8]

Kate's three-day campus visit spawned a lifetime of generosity to the Berry School. Whereas Alice gave with her heart and hands, Kate made numerous large financial contributions that enabled Martha

Berry to significantly expand her operation and to better meet the day-to-day needs of an ever-growing student body. She also established a $100,000 trust fund to provide Martha Berry with a private income. In addition, she influenced other women including her friend Emily Vanderbilt Sloane Hammond and Mrs. Andrew Carnegie to support the school. Emily Hammond and Martha Berry were introduced at Kate's home; subsequently, Mrs. Hammond became one of Miss Berry's most treasured friends. She is well-remembered for spearheading a "friends" organization, the Berry Pilgrims Association. Based in New York City and Westchester County, the "Pilgrims" met regularly and focused on fundraising from 1924 through the 1950s. Hammond regularly brought groups of friends on "pilgrimages" to the Berry School. Sara Delano Roosevelt (the mother of Franklin D. Roosevelt) and Mina Edison (Thomas Edison's widow) were among the well-known women who made the journey to Rome, Georgia.[9]

If we were to make a pilgrimage to Berry today we would find a 27,000-acre green campus that is the home of a well-regarded state-of-the-art college offering undergraduate and master's degrees. From humble beginnings, Martha Berry, her friends, staff, and students slowly crafted an institution that serves more than 2,000 young men and women from around the world. As in Kate's day, students continue to enrich their academic studies with on-campus work experience. Despite the many changes that would have been unimaginable to Kate, her direct contributions to the existing campus are quite significant. Among them are red brick Lemley Hall opened in 1921 as a boys' dormitory, "Macy" Memorial Library, which Kate donated to memorialize her sister-in-law Edith Carpenter Macy, and the Road of Remembrance built to honor Berry students who lost their lives in World War I. After the death of Martha Berry's mother, Kate assumed the cost of the extensive renovation of Berry's family home "Oak Hill" and the surrounding gardens; this allowed Miss Berry to entertain visitors in a genteel style. Today the 170-acre estate's historic home and history museum are open to the public. An oil portrait of Kate, which graced the entrance of Natirar during the convalescent home era, is displayed at the museum. In appreciation for her tremendous generosity and influence, Berry School recognized Kate, along with Emily Vanderbilt Hammond and Martha Berry, as an honorary member of the "The Daughters of Berry," an organization that Miss Berry founded in 1939 to preserve the traditions and heritage of her beloved school and home.

Kate's influence and support of Berry did not come to an end when she died. The Ladd Health Center is the most recent example of an important Ladd funded structure on campus; the money for the project was provided through the Kate Macy Ladd Fund. Currently, all student health and wellness services are located within The Ladd Center and include basic health and counseling services. Given Kate's personal struggles with poor health and her interest in medical philanthropy, it is an especially fitting representation of her largesse. The twenty-two-bed facility was dedicated on June 24, 1967.

"A $400,000 student health center of Georgian design sponsored by a Newark fund has been opened on the campus of Berry College…The new structure, a combination hospital and clinic, will provide Berry students with virtually every type of medical treatment except major surgery."[10]

Following the sale of Natirar to the King of Morocco in 1983, Berry College received a bequest of more than seven million dollars from Walter Ladd's estate as directed by his 1932 will.

Chapter 28

AS WE HAVE LEARNED FROM 1915 THROUGH 1917, Kate maintained a feverish pace of activity; Alice was almost always by her side. By this time Kate's health was far from perfect—she endured painful appendix and kidney issues, and in the hands of an assortment of doctors she was made to undergo hours of exploratory procedures and x-rays. The doctors concluded that although she had "an infected kidney and inflamed appendix and colitis" they were reluctant to operate. In that era, the removal of the appendix or a kidney was a frightening and potentially fatal proposition. Kate would have known about the death of her niece Elsie Ladd's fiancée during an appendectomy at his home in London several years before. Therefore, she accepted her fate and showed grit and resilience even though she felt "miserable."[1] All the while she counted her blessings and managed to roll up her sleeves, and return to her charity work. At her lowest ebb, she managed to focus on the positive. In particular she contemplated the joy and gratitude that she felt toward Alice, later saying,

> Her devotion to me all these many years could not be expressed in words for no words can describe it. I can only say, it was a perfect friendship. We liked the same people, enjoyed the same kind of music, and were interested in the same books, never tired of each other yet were always together. She always took breakfast in my room... and when I was so ill, ate all her meals beside my bed, feeding me at the same time. So, in spite of the many hard things I have had in life, I have been rich in loving care and devotion.[2]

Kate must have been coping with her physical discomfort fairly well. Even though she and Walter went to Bar Harbor later than usual in the summer of 1916, they entertained quite a bit throughout the season. Kate gave two specials concerts at Eegonos; she hosted an event for more than one hundred guests in late August and in mid-

September, a week after enduring a painful dental procedure she held another concert to benefit the YWCA at her home. She and Comus spent September 9th with Alice at the bungalow at Shady Nook. When Walter preceded her to Natirar, she and Alice remained on the *Wenonah* enjoying themselves until mid-October. With news from the war in Europe looking bleaker by the day, they may have anticipated that the steam yacht's future lay with the U.S. Navy. In any event, Kate considered this to be her most perfect cruise; as fate had it, this would be the last time that she and Alice cruised together.

Despite the worry and distraction of the Great War, Kate and Alice tried to make the most out of life. They attended theater and the opera every week and Kate was proud of the fact that she could walk twenty-two blocks at a time along the wintry streets of Manhattan. On February 7, 1917, she and her "dear Chickadee" went to see *A Successful Calamity* at the Booth Theater. It was a witty comedy written by the up-and-coming young playwright and lyricist Clare Beecher Kummer, a great-niece of Harriet Beecher Stowe; Kate raved about the performance of leading man William Gillette. Three days later, the women enjoyed Camille Saint-Saens's *Samson and Delilah* at the Met. By then they both had developed terrible colds; nonetheless, they continued to take long walks and visit with friends. Kate was helping her old chum Helen Hitchcock prepare to launch what would become The New York Art Alliance when Alice's health unexpectedly worsened. We can best understand the sudden turn in events as Kate expressed them a dozen years later in the most lengthy, evocative and emotion-filled passages of her memoir.

> February 14, called Dr. Devol in to see "Chickadee," and he said she had better go to bed for twenty-four hours; that she has no fever and nothing to worry about. She was never again to get out of bed. February 15th. She was very ill and we called Dr. Alex Miller, the lung specialist, and he said she had a fighting chance, but she was a very ill woman. We had two nurses at once for her and later a third...I was so anxious about "Chickadee."[3]

Dr. Sam Lambert stopped by and diagnosed Kate with bronchitis; even though she was far from well she refused to put her needs before those of her dearest friend. Augusta Hope, a southern-born New York friend whom Kate had introduced to Martha Berry (she subsequently became a "Berry Pilgrim"), wrote to alert Miss Berry in Georgia,

Have you heard how very very ill our dear Miss Lemley is at the
St. Regis and how very sick Mrs. Ladd is also? Miss "L." has
double-pneumonia and is often unconscious. Mrs. Ladd has
bronchitis and is brokenhearted over Miss Lemley's condition as we
all are...Please join your prayers with ours for these two friends.[4]

In her memoir Kate recounted,

On February 20th, Dr. Devol came five times to see
"Chickadee," and Sam and Dr. Kast and Dr. Miller saw her every
day, sometimes twice a day, and Dr. Devol stayed all night.
"Chickadee" liked him very much and he was a great comfort to
her; also Lil McKeand who could not reach the St. Regis until
February 21. I was so glad to see her. February 23, I lost my voice
completely and they were afraid to let me see "Chickadee," as
they feared my condition would worry her. February 24th, early in
the morning, my precious "Chickadee" died—a terrible sorrow to
me and a great loss.[5]

Alice drew her last breath at 1 a.m. on Saturday, February 24,
1917, at the St. Regis Hotel on East Fifty-Fifth Street. According to
her certificate of death, "the chief and determining cause of death was
double lobar pneumonia."[6] She had recently celebrated her forty-
seventh birthday; she and Kate had spent the last twenty-five years
together, more than half of Alice's life. Funeral plans fell into place
quickly. Presumably, Walter and Lily took charge, in consultation
with Kate, who noted that Everit and Edith "had a house in Fifty-
Sixth Street that winter and as they were away, we moved
"Chickadee" there."[7] A brief funeral service was conducted at the
Macy house on Sunday, but Kate's doctors would not allow her to
attend citing her own severe illness. Kate felt in desperate need of her
brother's solace; however he was far away from home. The Macys
had just taken up residence at Jekyll Island, Georgia, traveling with
their friend Edwin Gould, Sr. Tragically, on the very day that Alice
died, Gould's son Eddie was killed in a hunting accident in the woods
at Jekyll, and Everit and Edith were unable to leave the shocked and
bereft friends.

Augusta Hope knew that Martha Berry would wish to be of some
help to Kate, and she kept her well informed as events unfolded in
New York. She candidly wrote, "Mrs. Ladd is calm and lovely but
looks like a stricken flower. Mr. Ladd shows great emotion for once
in his life."[8] Kate was not allowed to accompany her dear

Chickadee's body home to West Chester, Pennsylvania for burial at Greenmount Cemetery. Her memories of this terrible episode never completely faded.

> The St. Regis people were all very kind and let me have my "Chickadee" beside me until the night before the funeral...everyone said it was a very sweet service. Dr. Slattery officiated. Sam and Dr. Kast showed wonderful judgment in letting me think I could go to the funeral. I even had my dress and hat made for I dressed in as deep mourning as I did for my own sister. She (Alice) was everything to me, and my life has never been quite the same since.[9]

The West Chester *Daily Local News* reported on Alice's funeral, stating that "so many flowers were sent here that a special car was required in conveying them through the borough."[10] From her desolate perch in New York City, all Kate could do was send an overwhelming array of floral arrangements as her final goodbye to her "Chickadee." While her friend Adelaide McAlpin Pyle stayed by her side and read the funeral service to her, Walter represented her at Alice's graveside, along with Lily Lemley McKeand and Augusta Hope, who commented that she had never seen more flowers at any funeral. A few hours after Alice was laid to rest Augusta wrote to tell Miss Berry that "a huge bouquet of pink roses tied with wide satin ribbon 'From Students and Faculty of the Berry School' was placed at Miss Lemley's feet." Martha Berry told Miss Hope that she was planning to include an article about Alice in the next edition of the *Berry School News,* and she requested the names and addresses of Alice's friends and family who would be interested in receiving a copy of the paper.[11]

Kate's use of the endearment "Chickadee" is quite touching; it is hard to know at what point in their relationship Kate bestowed this personal pet name upon Alice. The Chickadee was the darling of the bird world and groups were known to have congregated in Central Park in the 1890s. Bird lovers observed them to be diminutive yet feisty and energetic. Homage was paid to the tiny creatures in poetry and song and they were portrayed as inquisitive, confident, cheerful and faithful—all adjectives that Kate may well have used to describe Alice Lemley, her beloved Chickadee.

The weeks that followed Alice's premature death were

devastating to Kate who said, "I felt desperately lonely without dear 'Chickadee' and missed her at every turn." To make matters worse, she was fighting pneumonia and "forced to have two nurses." Kate remained in bed for five weeks; she did not leave the hotel until April 2. On April 6, her fifty-fourth birthday and the day that President Woodrow Wilson declared war against Germany, she returned to Natirar by private car. She described the house as seeming empty, but acknowledged that she had to "take up" her life and "learn to live a new life" with the strength that God gave her.[12]

As is often the case in the face of great loss, Kate found comfort by spending time with others who also cared deeply about Alice. Beulah Davis (a Lemley niece) joined Lil McKeand at Natirar where they spent three weeks going through Alice's things and recalling happy times. Lily also conducted business relative to her duties as her sister's executrix. Alice's will was probated in New Jersey and Maine that spring. Since the Ladds had always treated her with great generosity, she had amassed significant assets; it appears that Walter had managed her investments. Alice's securities were appraised at well over $25,000 (more than $480,000 in today's money) and her "Jewels, Chattels, Etc." included an assortment of watches, pearls, diamonds, stick pins, and brooches, most of which were gifts from Kate. In her will Alice requested that her 1915 pledge to "endow a day at Berry" be paid in full; the will also reflected her desire to bestow a few gifts to female friends including a parcel of land in Maine as well as cash. Otherwise, she bequeathed all of her money, personal effects, and the bungalow and its furnishings to Lily with the stipulation that it be passed on to their nieces in the future. A particularly poignant item that remains in the hands of a Lemley descendant is a Tiffany locket—an oval of onyx hanging from a chain of faceted black beads; the locket's smooth surface is embellished with the letters "KML" in gold. To this day, the piece is stored safely in its original black leather and satin-lined Tiffany case.

Throughout this period Kate considered ways to uphold Alice's memory. In recognition of her companion's interest in Berry College and her fondness for Martha Berry and the students Kate donated the "Lemley Hall" dormitory and she endowed funds for its furnishing and upkeep. Closer to home, Kate decided to create a memorial to aid the Visiting Nurse Association and the people it served; she knew that this would please Alice. As reported in the Raritan River Sub-Committee report for 1920-1921,

> The chief event of the year was the erection of an addition to the Nurse's Home in Peapack, built and furnished by Mr. and Mrs. Water G. Ladd in memory of Miss Alice Lemley. This addition consists of a reception room, recovery room, accommodating three beds and three cots and a bathroom. These, with the operating room form a wing with front and rear entrance entirely separate from the living quarters of the house, adding greatly to the efficiency of the clinic service as well as the liveableness of the home. A small sleeping porch at the rear of the house has been another much appreciated improvement.

> The "Alice Lemley Memorial" is so completely equipped that it could be used for a small General Hospital. It was opened to the public by a reception on October 20, 1920, but before this it had been used for three clinics.

> Through the co-operation of the Somerset Hills Garden Club and Mr. and Mrs. Ladd, the old out-buildings have been removed, the grounds put in order and beautified by a number of ornamental shrubs.[13]

A bronze plaque affixed to the front of the building made it clear that the state-of-the-art home and "hospital" were a tribute to Alice's dedication to her profession and to her commitment to the Visiting Nurse Association.

Chapter 29

ALICE'S PASSING LEFT A HOLE IN KATE'S HEART that ran deep and wide. After 1917, her memoir shifts in tone and becomes less illuminating; at times she is unusually preoccupied with her health. Perhaps the lack of depth and color as well as her self-absorption reflect her state of mind as she attempted to re-center her life.

At the very least, Kate felt satisfied knowing that the projects that meant so much to her and Alice continued to flourish. Maple Cottage was thriving under the direction of Estelle Dudley who patriotically oversaw the preparation of meals approved by the experts of the U.S. Food Administration to aid the war effort. Women were instructed to bake corn, oat, and barley bread in place of wheat, which was needed in Europe to feed "companions in arms and suffering women and children" and to prepare meatless dishes such as "Baked Hominy and Cheese" and "Bean Loaf" to insure adequate supplies of beef for "our own men and the men of our allied armies."[1]

The Visiting Nurse Association of the Somerset Hills also flourished as it serviced thousands of residents annually and increased fundraising efforts. Although Kate's previously vibrant involvement in her monthly V.N.A. meetings dwindled, she continued to play an important role as a trustee and major financial supporter and she maintained her interest in the success of the Peapack Nurse's Home until it was sold to a local physician in 1929.

As she managed her grief, Kate acknowledged what she called her husband's "devotion" as well as the kindness of her many loving friends, including female friends who had been mainstays throughout her life: Adelaide McAlpin Pyle, Dora Van Wyck Schenk, and Marie Ely Hill, and her sister-in-law Rebe. In addition, Kate was grateful for the unusual degree of attention she received from her newest physician, Ludwig Kast. Dr. Kast and Kate became acquainted in 1915 when he was caring for her brother. At that time both Everit and Alice had expressed full confidence in the physician's ability, which assured Kate to such an extent that before long he was in charge of all matters relative to her health. As she convalesced in the weeks after Alice died she recalled,

> Dr. Kast almost breathed for me, watching me almost hourly with the greatest tenderness and consideration. My brother once said, "Nothing you could possibly do for Dr. Kast could repay him for all his care..." No son could have done more, or been more thoughtful of me at this sad time and in the many hard ways which followed.[2]

With Alice's absence still looming large, Kate invited the doctor to join her and Walter at Bar Harbor; he accepted the invitation but lodged in the village with friend and fellow physician Edmund Devol rather than at Eegonos. It is clear that by the summer of 1917, Kast was well on his way to fully inserting himself into Kate's life.

> Dr. Kast was often in for lunch. He would come up and read amusing stories...and on July 30th brought up a case of live bees so I could watch them develop and come out...By August I was well enough to go to the Building of the Arts concerts. Dr. Kast nearly always went with us, getting a stool for my feet...[3]

That fall, Kast spent many days at Natirar, and Kate took him to visit with the women at Maple Cottage. Not long thereafter, when Kate returned to the St. Regis (her first time back since Alice died) she was greeted by a "helpful note" and lovely flowers from her physician and he came to visit her right away. Kast spent Christmas with the Ladds at Natirar because he felt that Kate's first Christmas "without dear 'Chickadee'" would be a lonely one. Throughout the months ahead, he continued to fuss over Kate, attending to her health and bearing lovely gifts.[4] During the summer of 1919, he stayed at Westover, on the Cleftstone Road at Bar Harbor; it is likely that the Ladds paid for the lease of the cottage. Kate reported that it was a good and busy season—she attended concerts, plays, and her YWCA meetings and entertained a constant stream of friends and family. When she hosted a musical that September, Dr. Kast was on hand to help her arrange the room. Upon her return to Natirar, she found that *Autumn Leaves From Maple Cottage,* the first of two delightful little books of inspiration that she and Kast had composed together had been printed. The books were ready to be given out as gifts to her guests at Maple Cottage, and she said that she did not think she was ever more thrilled in her life.[5]

At Dr. Kast's insistence, the Ladds gave up their apartment at the St. Regis; he maintained that the heating system was not good there. Kate was reluctant to do this because she always felt closest to Alice at the St. Regis, but she and Walter moved over to the Plaza as Kast advised. He coddled Kate, arriving for visits with food prepared by his own cook and chided her when she went out to see Heifetz perform on a wintry day. She climbed a flight of stairs and when Kast visited that night he told her that her kidney "dropped in his hand."[6] He warned her that with too much activity she would "keep on having attacks" until she would suffer an attack that she would not get over.[7]

Dr. Ludwig Walther Kast was poised to become a powerful influence on Kate's thinking about philanthropy. Even though he was a constant in her life for more than two decades she knew but a smattering of details about his personal history. He was not typical of members of her chosen circle, and beyond having a medical degree he had little in common with her previous physicians including S. Weir Mitchell and Winfield Scott Schley, patricians with fine American pedigrees like her own.

Kast was born in or near Vienna in 1877; his father was the Surgeon-General of the Austrian army and of Jewish ancestry. It is likely that the family had renounced their religious identity by the early twentieth century to protect themselves from the perils of anti-Semitism.[8] The men in the family were well-educated professionals; Kast followed in his father's footsteps and pursued a career in medicine. He commenced his studies at the University of Vienna in 1898 and received a medical degree in Prague six years later. Subsequently, he conducted research and furthered his studies in Leipzig and Berlin, which probably led to his invitation to join the staff of the Rockefeller Institute for Medical Research in New York City. Founded by John D. Rockefeller, Sr. in 1901, the new institution's purpose was to support medical research related to the prevention and treatment of disease.[9] Kast's education and experience in medical research made him attractive to the fledgling Rockefeller Institute. His native language was German; if he did not already possess English proficiency when he arrived in the United States in 1906, he quickly mastered the language.

Kast's tenure at the Rockefeller Institute was surprisingly brief. By 1907, he was an instructor in medicine at the New York Post-Graduate Medical School and Hospital; within a year he was also one of two associate editors of *The Post-Graduate,* the school's monthly journal of medicine and surgery. He encountered swift success at the medical school and was appointed to an assistant professorship in 1909. He became a full-professor in 1914. Kast simultaneously launched a consulting practice geared toward an upper-class clientele at 771 Madison Avenue, a stone's throw from Central Park and its fashionable residences, and he married, probably for the second time. A "Mrs. Kast" had accompanied him from Hamburg in 1906 but she was no longer in the picture by 1910. At about this time he wed Eugenie Clarissa Guenther, born in Milwaukee to a German father and Austrian mother. All seemed to be going exceedingly well for Ludwig Kast. He and his wife traveled to Europe in 1911 and spent the summer of 1912 in Paris. In March 1915, he became a naturalized citizen of the United States. However, by the following year, Eugenie was no longer involved in his activities and sometime after 1915 she returned to her family in Chicago where she spent the rest of her life.

We see that in less than a decade Ludwig Kast had managed to achieve citizenship and an enviable degree of success in his adopted country. Dark-haired, six feet tall and lanky, and only in his thirties when he and Kate met, Dr. Kast cleverly maneuvered his way into society. All the while he continued his affiliation with the New York Post-Graduate Medical School and worked to build an exclusive private practice. Kate called him "a very unusual man with great poise and understanding," and chances are good that he was aware of his charm.[10] Kast proved to be an adept man about town. He entertained his friends in the city and even hosted a group for a weekend of music, moonlight skating, and skiing at Yama Farms Inn, a well-known and exclusive Catskill Mountain retreat frequented by titans of industry, writers, musicians, and scientists. Margaret Woodrow Wilson, the president's eldest daughter was among Kast's guests who were photographed by "movie" men as they frolicked outdoors.[11] The physician joined the Grolier Club and the Harvey Scientific Society and served on the Endowment Committee at the Post-Graduate Medical School, working to convince potential donors, including James C. Brady and Vincent Astor, to make leading contributions to the school's endowment fund. Kast's combination of intelligence, European charm, and ease in society held him in good stead as he entered Kate's world. He would use these powers to influence her thinking and ultimately define both his legacy and hers.

Chapter 30

For many years, Kate and Walter planned to establish themselves as philanthropists through the creation of what they called the "Macy-Ladd Foundation." They drafted an initial certificate of incorporation as well as a set of bylaws in 1922; nonetheless, they never followed through with the incorporation of a joint foundation. The "official" explanation was that the couple's philanthropic goals had diverged.[1] Walter expressed an interest in supporting convalescent care as exemplified by Kate's success with Maple Cottage.[2] As she contemplated the future and the best use for her considerable fortune, Kate stepped away from the area of convalescence and focused on projects in the field of medical research, largely a result of long discussions with Ludwig Kast, although it also stands to reason that she might have been influenced by the Rockefellers' medical philanthropy. Although the Ladds' divergence of interests may seem natural on its face, a look beneath the surface is revealing.

Kate's dependence upon Ludwig Kast quickly deepened after Alice died. The year 1920 proved challenging for her. In December her appendix was finally removed, hardly optimal timing since Comus, Kate's comforting companion of fourteen years, had recently been put to sleep.[3] As she tried to recover from surgery under Dr. Kast's watchful eye, she also coped with perplexing and debilitating dental problems. Her teeth were repeatedly x-rayed; the clumsy equipment left her mouth aching and body exhausted. Over the course of the next few years, almost every one of her teeth would be extracted, including all four front teeth which were removed simultaneously. In addition, her jaw was operated on to remove bone fragments leading to the formation of abscesses. She felt certain that the routinely administered Novocain shots were poisoning her. Kate suffered along without appropriate pain medication or antibiotics. She ate pureed food like a baby and was fitted and re-fitted with "plates," which were never fully satisfactory. One dentist claimed that the plates would always pinch her due to the peculiar shape of the roof of her mouth.

Throughout this period, Dr. Kast remained Kate's chief confidant—amiable, devoted, sensitive, and thoughtful at every turn.

At times, he appears to have usurped Walter's role as Kate's husband and Walter took notice. According to a former Ladd employee he was indignant about Kast's influence over his wife and said that "he wanted desperately to have power over Kast and tried in every way to tie him up."[4] Rather than demand that Kate dismiss Kast, he gambled that by treating the doctor generously, the man would be in Walter's debt and come to depend upon him and that this would make it possible for Walter to control him. Walter bought Kast an expensive automobile and a place at Bar Harbor. Possibly at Walter's suggestion, Kate set up a trust for Kast that provided him an income of $10,000 a year.[5]

As her physician "on retainer" and a man who monitored every aspect of Kate's welfare, one might reasonably expect that Kate's overall health would have improved under Dr. Kast's care. Before Alice died, we recall that she was a physically vigorous woman—walking, skating, swimming, and tobogganing, despite nagging kidney and appendix issues. To the contrary, by the early 1920s her physical stamina declined—she was plagued by respiratory problems, and she lost weight. Kast brought in a parade of medical specialists, and Kate probably enjoyed the attention, but her concern over the complex dynamic that was growing between her husband and her physician may have spurred bouts of anxiety. Kate's frequent "helpful" conversations with Kast are the extent to which she received mental health counseling, and even though Kast served as the good doctor, standing by with a new medication or vaccine, it does not appear that he tried to help Kate regain enough physical strength to walk unassisted; if anything, he warned her against "overdoing it" and injuring her kidney beyond repair.

Even as Kate struggled to gain in health people close to her struggled as well. Ironically, her active and robust sister-in-law Edith Carpenter Macy suffered a fatal heart attack while vacationing with friends in Florida; everyone who knew her was stunned by the news. Kate was primarily concerned about her brother's well-being; he had always relied heavily upon his wife and was adrift without her. Two years later, Walter's brother William and his wife Elizabeth died within one month of each other. Far more tragically, Kate's sister-in-law Rebe Serrill Ladd took her own life. "My precious Rebe died suddenly; a terrible shock. No words can express all I feel, or how I shall miss her."[6] Kate had been concerned about the state of Rebe's mental health for years and tried repeatedly to intervene on her behalf. When James Ladd met with Kate at Natirar a few years before his wife died she recalled that Jim had upset her very much and he "misunderstood that I only wanted to help Rebe, for I foresaw trouble ahead for her. She is a great sufferer, and my heart is heavy about her for she is so dear to me."[7]

Despite her heartache, Kate repeatedly demonstrated her resilient nature. Rather than complain about her worries and discomforts she focused on her "red-letter" days and tried her best to maintain a sense of optimism about all things. She was busy assisting with projects to help Martha Berry, furnishing a new library for the pleasure of her Maple Cottage guests, and along with Walter she commissioned a magnificent series of stained glass windows in commemoration of their parents and Alice Lemley for the nave at St. Bernards Episcopal Church in Bernardsville. Kate also worked with Mabel Smith Douglass, dean of The New Jersey College for Women (a branch of Rutgers University, which had been founded in 1918). She donated "Willets Infirmary," a state-of-the-art campus medical building in memory of her sister Mae. In 1925, in recognition of her interest and support of women's health and education, Dean Douglas went to Natirar and presented Kate with a "diploma of Master of Arts."[8] The Willets infirmary continues to provide women's health and wellness services on the campus of what is now known as Douglass College.

Although we cannot pinpoint the exact date, records suggest that between 1926 and 1927, while wintering in California, Dr. Kast wrote to Kate and proposed that she start a medical foundation, something that they could work on and watch grow together. He further indicated that he had received a job offer in California, a job he felt that he would have to accept it if Kate did not agree to his foundation plan. The possibility of losing Kast in an instant was more than Kate could bear. Without consulting Walter, she agreed to his proposal. Is it possible that Kast fabricated the offer of a job in California to push Kate to accept his plan? The answer to this question is unknown, but Walter Ladd was so disturbed over this fast turn of events that according to one of his employees, he was "beyond words and never forgave Kast."[9]

The following year, Walter was still feeling displeased about the situation that Kast had set in motion. In addition, even though eighteen months had passed, he had not fully recovered from a serious riding accident. Perhaps he compensated for his sense of irritation to some degree when he decided to pursue one of his great personal dreams—he commissioned the firm of Cox and Stevens to design a stunningly elegant schooner to be built to his specifications in Kiel, Germany, an important naval port in the Baltic Sea.

In contrast, the year 1928 found Ludwig Kast on top of the world. In February he married Marie Schultz Aufermann, a widow who lived nearby on Park Avenue. One might have expected Kate to feel a tinge of jealousy toward the bride; however, it appears that the marriage genuinely pleased her. She commented, "Dr. Kast has brought a new joy into my life, for I know I shall love Marie."[10] Hours after their wedding ceremony the newlyweds motored out to see Kate; she said that she would never forget the joy their visit brought her. The Kasts spent the winter in California, and when they came home they rushed to be with Kate at Natirar. She wrote, "If I had a son, who had married, his wife could not have been sweeter with me in every way; so thoughtful and loving; in fact, it seemed as if she had brought me new life, and to see my dear Dr. Kast's happiness seems all I could ask."[11] In June, Kate increased Kast's annual income to $25,000 per year.[12] This large increase probably coincided with his new role—at Kate's "request" he carried out a survey of organized philanthropy to learn where other foundations concentrated their support. The survey revealed promising opportunities for philanthropic efforts in the larger field of medicine and health, "where there appears to be an urgent need for integration of knowledge and practice." Kast determined that most medical and public health research was funded by educational institutions, which focused on biochemistry and physiology as opposed to the fields of psychobiology and sociology. Based on his findings, he suggested that Kate establish a foundation to fill the existing gap and "promote human welfare through assistance to scientific medicine and improved healthcare."[13]

While Kate and Dr. Kast worked to sharpen the focus of Kate's intended philanthropy, Walter focused his energy on every aspect of his new yacht's design and furnishing. It is likely that Walter felt a sense of urgency due to both his age, and to the understanding that his long-held financial arrangement with Kate was about to end.[14]

Perhaps as a nod to his wife, who was the source of his financial independence, he christened his yacht *Etak*. In any event, in 1929, with the public reeling from the aftermath of "Black Tuesday" and a price tag exceeding $350,000, *Etak* may well have been viewed as a lavish and frivolous example of conspicuous consumption and perhaps an old man's final fling. Nevertheless, the Ladds could afford such an extravagance. Kate's personal secretary Phoebe Edgar said that after the stock market crash, they had just as much money as ever. She believed that their combined assets amounted to approximately forty-six million dollars.[15] As the finishing touches were being put on *Etak*, Kate was occupied quietly at home writing her memoir, *The Story of My Life*. It was published by Mosher Press of Portland, Maine (the company that had previously produced her books for Maple Cottage), and printed, bound, and delivered that winter.

As she drafted her memoir Kate welcomed a constant stream of visitors to Natirar including her brother and the Kasts. She noted that she and Kast had "helpful" conversations, reminiscent of her intimate talks with Rebe and Dr. Mitchell. She also wrote that Everit was "very bloated" but "cheerful," and said that he was "so dear and we had some lovely talks."[16] It is likely that Kate's plan for a medical philanthropy was among the things they discussed.

Close friends and family members were aware that after 1915 Everit frequently suffered from poor health and, like Kate, was prone to spells of depression that bordered on mental and physical breakdown. His wife had always taken over when he was having difficulties, and those who knew him best observed that after Edith died, Everit's characteristic drive had diminished.[17] Two days before Christmas 1929, Everit underwent what Kate called "a big sinus operation," which left her feeling especially anxious.[18] Since he had suffered with chronic sinus problems for years, as a widower, Everit wintered in Arizona. Early in 1930, he traveled to Phoenix with his secretary as well as his longtime butler William Halkett. Although his health was compromised, he was not considered dangerously ill. Therefore, Kate was completely shocked to receive word of her brother's death on March 21, 1930, two days before what would have been his fifty-ninth birthday. Six days later, a funeral service was held at Chilmark, his New York estate. Microphones were installed to carry the voices of the officiating clergymen and choir across the Hudson River to Natirar so that Kate could follow the funeral of her closest and most beloved relative quietly in the privacy of her home.[19]

There is some speculation that Everit's sudden passing accelerated the announcement of Kate's new foundation. Behind the scenes, Kate's advisors and Dr. Kast drafted bylaws and articles of incorporation. On the heels of her brother's untimely death, there was discussion regarding the name of the burgeoning foundation; among those considered were the Josiah and Everit Macy Foundation and the Josiah-Everit Macy Foundation. In the end, Kate simply named the foundation to honor her father, Josiah Macy Jr., perhaps because it was his fortune that made her significant wealth possible.

According to her secretary's sworn testimony, Kate had asked Walter to "set up" the Foundation on her behalf but he refused to do it—Kate wanted him to select securities from her portfolio to be transferred to her newly incorporated philanthropy. When he was unwilling to cooperate, Kate instructed a favorite nurse, Madeline McCue, to telephone W. R. Reed, Walter's secretary, and ask him to start to identify stocks for the transfer. Two days later Walter went to his office and began to choose stocks from lists that Mr. Reed had drawn up.[20] Dave Hennen Morris, Kate's attorney and the husband of her friend Alice Vanderbilt, was her legal representative. He was personally interested in moving things along quickly so that he could depart for Europe toward the end of April. Fifteen founding directors were listed in the "Certificate of Incorporation of the Josiah Macy Jr. Foundation." Among them were Kate's nephews, Noel and Valentine Macy Jr. and Josiah Macy Willets as well as Ludwig Kast (who would serve as the foundation's first president), Chairman of the Board Dave Morris and both his son and son-in-law. Noticeably absent from the board was Walter Ladd.

On April 24, 1930, Kate officially established the Josiah Macy Jr. Foundation with an initial gift of five million dollars. With prescient wisdom she outlined her intentions for the Josiah Macy Jr. Foundation in her letter of gift,

> It is my desire that the Foundation in use of this gift should concentrate on a few problems rather than support many undertakings, and that it should primarily devote its interest to fundamental aspects of health, of sickness, and of methods for the

relief of suffering. To these ends, the Foundation might give preference in the use of this fund to integrating functions in medical sciences and medical education for which there seems to be particular need in our age of specialization and technical complexities. Believing as I do, that no sound structure of social or cultural welfare can be maintained without health, that health is more that freedom from sickness, that it resides in the wholesome unity of mind and body, I hope that your undertaking may help to develop more and more in medicine, in its research and the ministry of healing the spirit which sees the center of all its efforts in the patient as an individuality. I hope therefore that the Foundation will take more interest in the architecture of ideas than in the architecture of buildings and laboratories.[21]

The announcement of the new Foundation appeared immediately in the New York press where Ludwig Kast commented that the trustees had no definite plans for the Foundation, but they expected to set to work planning things out right away. This underscores the haste with which news of the organization was unveiled.[22] Walter did not appear to share his wife's excitement. It has been suggested that he was absent from New York in April 1930, heading to Kiel to christen and take possession of his new schooner. A photograph taken in Germany on the deck of *Etak* in early May shows an elderly man, who resembles Walter, sharing a toast with the yacht's crew. Walter Ladd probably accompanied them on *Etak's* maiden voyage. She docked in New York on May 30, 1930, having been twenty-eight days at sea.[23]

The board of directors quickly realized that Kate was far more than a generous woman with deep pockets—she showed wisdom and vision and "unflagging interest" in the work of the foundation until the end of her life.[24]

By the time the Macy Foundation trustees gathered for their first annual meeting at the home of Chairman Dave Morris on East Seventieth Street in New York City, concrete plans to fund initial projects were underway. Although Kate was not in attendance that evening she expressed her appreciation to the board by sending flowers with a gracious note to say that she would be with them in thought.[25] The trustees passed a number of resolutions including the appropriation of $1,250 to Professor Albert Einstein to provide a fellowship for a research assistant.[26] The following day *The New York*

Times reported that Dave Morris had met with Einstein in Germany the previous summer—the scientist had mentioned that he was having difficulty financing his research. Morris conveyed Dr. Einstein's need of funds to the Foundation, and the board voted to cover "all the expenses of a famous German mathematician capable of helping Dr. Einstein toward quicker solution of the scientific secrets which he seeks to fathom."[27] *TIME Magazine* elaborated, "Last week, the Josiah Macy Jr. Fund, created six months ago by Mrs. Walter Graeme Ladd (of the rich New Jersey Macy family), established a fellowship to pay the expense of an assistant for Dr. Einstein. First incumbent will be his good friend and familiar, Dr. Walter Mayer, mathematician at the University of Vienna."[28] It may seem odd that one of the Foundation's first grants funded nonmedical research, a fellowship that made it possible for Walter Mayer to work on an investigation into the fundamental laws of physics. However, a history of the Macy Foundation explains that due to the economic depression of the late 1920s and 1930s there was a reduction in the funding of scientific research. This circumstance led the foundation to occasionally extend "emergency aid." It was further noted that Ludwig Kast and Albert Einstein were friends.[29] With their common ancestry, native language, scientific training, and concern about conditions in Europe where both men had friends and relatives in danger, Drs. Kast and. Einstein made for well-suited companions.[30]

Perhaps another unstated reason that the Macy Foundation assisted Dr. Einstein was simply because it would have been difficult to resist involvement with a man of his renown; by 1930, Einstein was a cultural icon. The American public was charmed by the shaggy-haired disheveled genius; his tremendous celebrity could only garner positive publicity for the fledgling foundation. On December 10, 1930, Einstein and his colleague Walter (Walther) Mayer arrived in New York, en route to California via the Panama Canal on the Red Star Line's *S.S. Bergenland*. Newspapers as diverse as *The New York Times, The Danville Bee* (Virginia), and *The Evening Huronite* (South Dakota) covered the story of the brilliant scientist who cherished his privacy. To this end, his public appearances were kept to a minimum, and he never appeared for the purpose of self-promotion. For example, while in New York City he spoke (in German) on behalf of several Jewish organizations and attended a luncheon hosted by legendary publisher Adolph Ochs of *The New York Times* before departing for Pasadena. A few months later Ludwig Kast and his wife Marie joined Albert and Elsa Einstein for the first of several winter get togethers in southern California where Einstein was being courted by the California Institute of Technology.

Much as Kast was pleased to have helped his friend with an allocation from the foundation, Kate was enthusiastic about allocations in a new area of medicine that addressed the interplay of mind and body in the function of the whole human being. Kate was well-acquainted with the effect that anxiety and depression could have on physical function. As we have learned she and her brother Everit both experienced bouts of "melancholy," which directly affected their health and well-being. Her interest in what later came to be known as the mind-body connection took root early in the twentieth century when she and Alice first dabbled in the religious "mental-healing movement," and consulted with a popular spiritualist Lenora Piper in Montclair, New Jersey. In 1931, her interest in how emotions and attitudes affected health and the treatment of disease took center stage when she personally and "energetically supported" the selection of Dr. Helen Flanders Dunbar, the pioneering twentieth century American psychiatrist, psychoanalyst, and pastoral counselor, as the recipient of a Macy Foundation grant for an investigation of the existing literature on the relationship between emotions and disease. With the 1935 publication of Dunbar's massive book, *Emotion and Bodily Changes,* the Macy Foundation made a groundbreaking contribution to the new field of psychosomatic medicine.[31] In 1939, the first volume of the journal *Psychosomatic Medicine* was published with financial assistance from the foundation and under the editorship of Dr. Dunbar.[32]

Kate's ideas continued to carry significant weight with the foundation; in May 1931 she suggested that the foundation support a study of migraines, research on the cause of arteriosclerosis and the general topic of aging, and a review of schools that offered programs for the study of professional social work in the United States and Canada. Kate gave regular monetary gifts to the foundation to acknowledge her appreciation for the board's good work and to help ensure that her pet projects would be pursued. On April 6, 1932, her sixty-ninth birthday, she wrote to Kast and sent a gift to mark the second anniversary of the creation of the Josiah Macy Jr. Foundation, indicating that she was "much interested in the report of progress in the affairs of the Foundation." She asked him to convey to the Board her appreciation and "deep sense of gratitude for their wise stewardship..." She also requested that by adding her latest contribution to her previous gifts she hoped that the trustees would soon approve "projects concerning the social aspects of medicine."[33]

Between 1930 and 1941, the year that Ludwig Kast died and the reigns of leadership were turned over to Dr. Willard C. Rappleye, the Josiah Macy Jr. Foundation allocated about $1.5 million to research projects, primarily to fund studies of interest to Kate.

Chapter 31

As the Josiah Macy Jr. Foundation began to hit its stride, Kate's and Walter's personal lives were moving along more slowly. By the standards of the day, they were an elderly couple. While life together was never a fairytale, their marriage endured for almost fifty years. We know that Kate always regretted her childless state, but fortunately relationships with the youngsters of friends and her nieces and nephews helped to fill the void as she aged. Although, according to one of Kate's great-nieces, Walter was never interested in children, a glimpse at photos from the early 1930s shows Kate and Walter on the patio at Eegonos looking every bit like a pair of kindly grandparents: a snowy-haired Kate beams and cradles one of her brother's infant grandchildren in her arms.[1]

By the late 1920s Kate was known to refer to her favorite nurses as "her girls" and she was particularly fond of one of them, Roberta "Ruby" Catherine Firlotte. As Kate recalled, "On August 18, 1926, I saw and engaged dear little Miss Firlotte, who was to be one of my greatest comforts for years to come. A sweet quiet, capable little woman and most unselfish."[2]

Kate treated Ruby like a daughter. The young woman had been raised by relatives in New Brunswick, Canada while her single mother worked as a housekeeper in Maine. At some point, Ruby joined her mother and attended high school in Bar Harbor. Her actual nurse training was rudimentary, and according to her grandson, she was more Kate's companion than nurse and viewed "Mrs. Ladd" as a mother figure.[3] Knowing that Ruby had a meager childhood, Kate tried to make up for it by giving her luxuries that she could never have afforded including an expensive civit fur coat and opportunities for travel. When the young woman was in an accident and required a small operation, Kate fussed over her like a mother hen. While in New Jersey with Kate, Ruby met Nicholas Meany, a local Bernardsville man, and a serious romance ensued. "Rubbles" and

"Nickie" maintained an avid correspondence filled with poignant declarations of love and longing for more than a year. After he visited Eegonos, for what amounted to an audience with Kate, Ruby wrote and said, "Mrs. Ladd has been talking of you all afternoon. She is most happy and feels that you are just the man she would pick out for me—I can't imagine anyone saying anything better."[4]

With her engagement secured, Ruby was eager for Kate (whom she would always referred to as "Mrs. Ladd") to assume the role of "mother-of-the-bride." The preoccupation of wedding planning did wonders for Kate as it helped to offset her continued sorrow over Everit's death as well as her concern over his three children, each of whom was experiencing marital difficulties that would lead to divorce. Her desire to ensure that Ruby would have a storybook wedding day filled a special need for Kate at a time when she was feeling somewhat adrift. Both Walter and Ludwig Kast were pre-occupied. Kast had jumped head-on with the Foundation and was making plans that would include squiring Dr. Einstein around in California in the months ahead. Walter was busy with his newly acquired dream yacht, and he may have showed signs of being smitten with the young nurse who had cared for him during his convalescence in Thomasville, Georgia, where he had gone to recover from the aftereffects of his riding injuries.

On August 26, 1930, Ruby and Nick exchanged vows during a high nuptial mass at the Catholic Church of the Holy Redeemer in Bar Harbor. The local newspaper, *The Bar Harbor Times* called it "one of the most brilliant ever to take place in Bar Harbor. The church was completely filled with relatives and friends."[5] Among the guests were many of the Ladds' personal friends and employees, including the Morrises and Lil and David McKeand who were staying at the Shady Nook bungalow that Lil had inherited from Alice. The newspaper described Ruby's bridal gown as a "superb gown of ivory satin worn more than forty years ago by Mrs. Walter Graham Ladd."[6] In actuality, Ruby did not wear Kate's original wedding dress; the gown was more of a hybrid that incorporated but a small bit of Kate's 1883 gown and in no way resembled the dress she wore when she and Walter wed. However, with her voluminous veil and train and bridal bouquet of white roses and lilies of the valley Ruby was a sight to behold. Her wedding portraits reveal a lovely bride along with an attractively outfitted wedding party—the men looking stylish in hired suits with identical waistcoats, striped pants, coats, cravats, and spats and the women wearing up-to-the-minute dresses of gold and aquamarine chiffon with matching hats and shoes. This degree of elegance would not have been typical for people of working class means, and hints at the degree of Kate's involvement. She also made it possible to hold a catered wedding lunch at the Parish Hall where palms and massive floral arrangements set a festive scene. Her generosity extended beyond the actual day of Ruby's marriage. Now that Walter had *Etak*, Kate gave the bride and groom a month-long honeymoon sailing cruise to Mexico and South America on the Ladds's smaller yacht, *Wenonah*, as a wedding gift along with a house in Summit, New Jersey. The Ladds' Natirar superintendent Stanley Jones, who attended the wedding with his wife Betty, had been instructed to remove furniture in storage at Natirar to help furnish Ruby and Nick's new home.

"Mrs. Ladd" and Ruby remained close throughout the rest of Kate's life, even after the Meanys and their young daughter moved to the Pacific Northwest where Nick worked in the lumber business. In 1934 Kate had decided to create trust funds for a number of people for whom she felt deep affection and Ruby was among them. As a result, the Meany family enjoyed the financial benefit of Kate's generosity throughout Ruby's lifetime. Her grandson confided that "Mrs. Ladd's" many acts of kindness toward Ruby made a profound difference for the well-being of his family, something he would never forget.

Much as Kate was comforted by her favorite nurse and companion, Walter found refuge in a relationship with another nurse, Florence Jones Vaughn, whose tenure overlapped that of Ruby Firlotte. Although they each hailed from towns that were known to cater to the rich, their backgrounds could not have been more dissimilar.

Florence Jones Vaughn was a southerner with a pedigree. She was a native of Thomasville, Georgia, which was known as a popular winter resort, especially attractive to the affluent sportsman. Her parents were first cousins and her paternal grandmother and maternal great-uncle had been raised just outside of town on the Jones family's 10,000-acre Greenwood Plantation. Miss Vaughn's paternal grandfather had been a revered Confederate General, further burnishing the family lineage; nevertheless, the Jones's fortunes had been irrevocably diminished in the aftermath of the Civil War. Despite this circumstance, Florence's parents remained prominent members of their community.

Prior to meeting Walter Ladd, Florence worked as a trained nurse. The pair met when she served as one of his private nurses during his stay in Thomasville in the winter of 1927. By this time the Jones and Vaughn families had given up their ancestral home and Greenwood Plantation had returned to its former glory in the hands of Oliver Payne, a treasurer of the Standard Oil Company. It was passed on to his descendants and was a prominent estate which would welcome social luminaries for decades. Even though she lived in a modest house in town, Florence must have made a positive impression on Walter; she was bright, cultured, and fairly young. After two months time, she was asked to accompany him north to continue to assist with his convalescence. Perhaps the lure of adventure convinced her to forsake her familiar, small-town life for what would have been a glamorous opportunity for a single working woman—although Walter was forty years her senior, he was wealthy and known to be generous and impulsive. It is difficult to surmise what Kate thought of Florence's sudden appearance at Natirar on April 15, 1927, although she did observe that her husband looked greatly improved. When Walter no longer required the services of a private nurse he appears to have been unwilling to dismiss Miss Vaughn, and she was assigned the role of housekeeper. In the final paragraph of her memoir Kate wrote,

> I must not finish my diary without saying a word about my two devoted nurses, Miss McCue and Miss Firlotte who have taken such excellent care of me for three years and been a great comfort to me. Miss Firlotte has been with me four years next summer and I have never known her to say an impatient word in all that time. Miss Vaughn has also taken all the household cares from me—a great help.[7]

We may be tempted to read between the lines since Kate hardly offers a ringing endorsement of her young housekeeper. Paul Smart (Adelaide McAlpin Pyle's son-in-law) was one of Walter's executors and he reported that prior to Walter's death "there had been generally in charge of the household a housekeeper but immediately following his death she was not employed further."[8]

It is telling that Kate wasted no time in sending Florence on her way but she felt assured that Florence would never face dire straits like so many Americans in the depth of the Depression. The thirty-five years old woman had a vocation; she returned to Thomasville and worked at the John D. Archbold Memorial Hospital (established in 1925 by the son of a Standard Oil operative in memory of his father). She lived in her parents' home, never married, and worked until the end of her life, even though she could easily have afforded to retire thanks to the generosity of her former employer—Walter had bequeathed her the sum of $25,000 (roughly $480,000 in today's money) which was a significantly greater amount of money than he had provided for any other employee including his long-standing estate superintendent. In contrast to Ruby Meany, who lived until 1983, always surrounded by a loving family, Florence Vaughn's life was less enviable. In 1970, she died at Archbold Memorial, the hospital where she worked for most of her nursing career, leaving no immediate heirs.

As we have learned, during the period when Florence was in residence at Natirar and Bar Harbor, Walter was struggling on several fronts. He was dealing with the effects of his injuries and the associated physical limitations, as well as the fallout with Kate and Kast over the Foundation, both circumstances that may have undercut his sense of manliness. In addition, he and his contemporaries were aging, and he faced the deaths of friends, his brother-in-law and his brothers William and Jim, and their wives, all in a relatively brief span of time.

Whereas Kate's focus was the Foundation and doing special things for family, friends, employees, and even strangers, Walter's chief enjoyment by the early 1930s was to spend time at Eegonos and on his yacht. He developed a friendship with Kate's cousin Nelson Macy who had been close to Everit in their younger years. He had served with the U.S. Navy in the Spanish American War, was a former president of the Navy League and, like Walter, a lifetime yachting enthusiastic and member of the New York Yacht Club. An engineer by training, his life was in transition in the early 1930s: He was newly retired, twice a widower, and recovering from an engagement that had abruptly fizzled. In Walter he found a companion with a similar passion for yachting. As the men enjoyed sailing together in the summer of 1932, no one could have predicted that their September cruise at Newport would be one of Walter's last hurrahs at sea.

Other than minor ailments and the injuries sustained during his riding accidents, Walter Ladd had been a relatively healthy and active man throughout his life. However, in May 1933, he took ill and on May 19 he was transported to Doctors Hospital in New York City. *TIME Magazine* called Doctors the "Richest Hospital." It boasted an array of opulent amenities typically found in first-class hotels including nourishment prepared by a French chef. All of the institutions' medical and surgical equipment was the most modern and efficient, and the professional staff was of the highest caliber.[9] Despite these advantages, on May 22, Walter succumbed to pneumonia after a brief stay. The New York and New Jersey newspapers provided perfunctory mention of his life of seventy-six years. He was remembered as a lawyer (incorrectly) and a yachtsman; much of his obituary was devoted to coverage of his wife's recent philanthropy. Items in the *Bar Harbor Times* were a bit more personal. He was described as one of the island's "oldest and most beloved" summer residents, a warden and longtime vestry member of St. Savior's Episcopal Church, and a generous and unostentatious contributor to the local YMCA.[10]

Walter's funeral service was held at the historic Grace Church in New York City. The rector of the church was assisted by Reverend T. A. Conover from St. Bernards Church where Walter was affiliated in New Jersey. Among his pallbearers were Macy family members including Kate's nephew Noel and her cousin William Kingsland Macy as well as longtime family friends such as William Hill, John D. Rockefeller, Jr., and Dave Morris. Like most members of the Macy family Walter was laid to rest at Woodlawn cemetery where Kate had purchased a 2,500 square foot burial plot for $10,000 in the Golden Rod section in 1919. It was just a short walk from the "Magnolia" section where the Macys had been interred since the late 1860s. However, the Ladds' final resting place was far more opulent than the humble Macy burial plot. It was designed by an up-and-coming architect and Macy family friend Eric Kebbon and featured a bas-relief decorated semi-circular granite wall. A pair of matching ledger stones edged with a palm leaf pattern marked the location of a 7.6-foot underground vault. According to the death certificate, like Alice Lemley, Walter succumbed to lobar pneumonia. The date of death written on the certificate was May 22, 1933, his gravestone shows the date May 21, 1933.

It seems likely that Kate was not in attendance either in New York City for her husband's funeral service or in the Bronx for his internment. At the time of his death Walter was making plans to close up the New Jersey property and open the Bar Home residence for the season. Kate elected to continue to Bar Harbor as planned in early June. In August she wrote to her nephew Noel, Everit's middle child, and his second wife Polly who were out west, as was his brother Valentine who had also remarried,

> You will be interested to know that Paul Smart has sold the *Etak* for me—when everyone told me there was no chance to sell her this year, as no one was buying boats. We only got $65,000 & she cost $364,886.29 but she cost me $10,000 a year just to keep her up, so I felt it a good thing to face our losses when we had a chance to get something. Kingsland's brother-in-law Adolph Dick bought her, and Uncle Walter was very fond of Julia & her family, and I am happy to know she will be used by friends.[11]

Kate said that she thought often of Walter when she first arrived at Bar Harbor that summer, surrounded as she was by water. She decided that the best thing for her to do was to turn her thoughts to memories of the happy days on their different yachts throughout the years. She would only occupy Eegonos for a few more summers. After Lil McKeand passed away in 1935, erasing her strongest connection to Alice, she stopped making her summer pilgrimage to Maine. It seemed as if she suddenly lost her taste for her beloved summer home.

Walter and Kate each filed a last will and testament on February 23, 1932, fifteen months before Walter died. Even though Walter never joined Kate in support of her Foundation, he also wished to see his fortune used in a thoughtful and meaningful way. After he died his net estate was valued at over eleven million dollars.[12] Through his will he made monetary and material bequests to family members, friends, and employees, and named his wife the life beneficiary of the entire residue of his estate. Kate received the benefit of his income and both properties and their contents for life. His will instructed that after his wife's death, the reminder of his estate be directed to provide legacies to several churches, hospitals, schools, and libraries, and most significantly to fund "Trust A." This would be administered by a corporation to be called the Kate Macy Ladd Fund. In all likelihood Walter had developed "Trust A" in consultation with Kate. Its intent was the creation and maintenance of a:

> Home in which deserving gentlewomen who are compelled to depend upon their own exertions for support shall be entertained without charge for periods of time while convalescing from illness, recuperating from impaired health, or otherwise in need of rest, in such numbers and at such times as available accommodations and the income assigned by such corporation to such trust will from time to time permit.[13]

The convalescent home was to be established in the mansion house at Natirar and operated for a period of fifty years dated from the time of Walter's death. Through the home's establishment Walter hoped to "insure the development and carry on the work which my beloved wife Kate Macy Ladd started in memory of her parents Josiah Macy Jr. and Caroline L. Macy, and which is now maintained and known as 'Maple Cottage.'"[14] He stipulated that the directors appointed to administer the Kate Macy Ladd Fund would be empowered to sell lands and property belonging to the Natirar estate as deemed expedient. Through the creation of the trust he acknowledged his wife's early successful healthcare advocacy for women at Maple Cottage. Perhaps it was a sign of his respect and admiration for Kate's pioneering efforts at Maple Cottage that his will directed that an oil portrait of Kate be displayed in the main room at Natirar once it had been transformed into the Kate Macy Ladd Convalescent Home. He further instructed that the portrait (painted by Adele Herter circa 1914) be transferred for display at the headquarters of the Josiah Macy Jr. Foundation in New York City upon termination of the trust. His wishes were followed explicitly.

Chapter 32

AS A WIDOW, KATE BLOSSOMED. Although she missed the husband who had been a dependable and familiar presence in her life over five decades, it does not appear that she grieved for him as deeply as she had mourned the loss of Alice Lemley. Within the year, Kate was forging new relationships and looking toward the future. Her resilience and positivity increased along with her continued desire to help others.

By the 1930s Kate had become known as a health advocate and philanthropist largely due to her creation of the Josiah Macy Jr. Foundation. She also made other significant charitable gifts in support of health. For example, in 1935 she contributed $35,000 to the United Hospital Campaign, a New York City charity, which supported public hospitals. She was singled out and praised in the newspaper as "the donor of the largest gift by an individual." The article explained that Kate had long been interested in hospital work and was stimulated to get involved after hearing that "the racketeers of New York took as their illegal tributes more than the voluntary hospitals were pleading for."[1] When the committee of the Visiting Nurse Service of the Henry Street Settlement announced the status of their annual fundraising campaign in *The New York Times*, it was noted that the second largest contribution came from Mrs. Ladd, "a friend of Miss Wald for many years," and in 1937 her name was again in the spotlight in an article that praised a second leading donation of $56,000 to the United Hospital Fund.[2] Kate's interest in politics, world conditions, and war-related developments in Europe inspired her to make a significant donation to the British Ambulance Corp in 1940 and she was proud that the Macy Foundation sponsored initiatives associated with national defense through the allocation of more than $650,000 to aid medical research and education directly involved with war-related issues including traumatic shock and war neurosis.[3] Of particularly far-reaching impact was a Foundation initiative designed to support medical professionals during wartime—a one-of-a-kind reprint service through which the Foundation distributed publications to U.S. military doctors. These publications made it possible for them to stay abreast of new developments in medical research and practice while serving with the armed forces. The program was so well received that it was expanded to send reprints to doctors serving with U.S. allies in Europe and Asia. Overall, more than six million copies of 400 medical and scientific papers and journal articles were distributed.[4]

While we know that Kate was raised in an altruistic family, it is fair to say that she elevated their example of "doing good" to an inspired height with her seemingly unlimited resources and tremendous capacity for generosity. Although medical philanthropy was the primary focus of her largesse, she never stinted on other charity work and was always ready to help family, friends, and acquaintances. Kate's smaller acts of kindness have become legendary, as noted by her secretary who compiled an imposing list of the donations and gifts Kate made between the years 1920 and 1945—many of these were sums in excess of $500 but thousands of gifts in lesser amounts were given as well. Miss Edgar suggested that

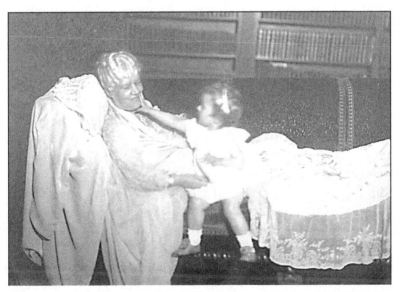

"Aunt Kate" and great niece Edith Carpenter Macy, circa 1929, in the Natirar Library (*Courtesy of Edith Macy Shoenborn*)

since her employer had so much money, she never felt the need for it. For example, when she inherited $400,000 from the estate of her aunt Mary Macy Kingsland who had died in 1919, she gave every penny away; her pleasure was to use her money to uplift others.[5]

Charming recollections abound regarding Kate's kindness and generosity toward family and staff. According to Miss Edgar, Kate always gave gifts to her employees. She sent one nurse on an all-expense-paid vacation and since it pleased the woman so much Kate gave seven or eight employees a gift of $1,000 (the equivalent of an $18,000 gift in 2017) to use toward their vacation of choice; Miss Edgar remarked that because she made the first person so happy Mrs. Ladd wanted to make others happy as well.[6] Kate took similar delight in helping her great-nieces Julia and Mary Willets when she provided them with money to rescue Rose Pinkham Macy's sterling silver tea pot from an antique dealer. The girls wanted to give it to their parents as a silver wedding anniversary gift; thanks to Kate's intervention the early nineteenth century teapot was returned to the Macy family. More than eighty years later the heirloom remains in the family in the possession of Julia's daughter. When Kate learned that her nephew Valentine's former wife Lydia Bodrero Macy was visiting France, she gaily presented the beautiful young woman with a check for $1,000 with the suggestion that she buy herself some hats in Paris; Lydia's daughter Edith has never forgotten her mother's surprise and joy. Kate's generosity and compassion even extended to the relatives of friends. Upon hearing that a granddaughter of her childhood friend Sally Whitcomb was suffering through the indignity of protruding teeth, she quietly covered the prohibitive expense of extensive orthodontic care, a gesture that resulted in a renewed sense of self-confidence for the girl for life.

Although her smaller acts of private giving may have meant the most to her, Kate's name was in the spotlight in the local press associated with social events as well as in connection with important philanthropic activities.

During her lifetime Kate had intentionally remained on the fringe of society, possibly due to some combination of her Quaker upbringing, her marriage to a man who did not have an upper-class background, and her general lack of interest in the world of high society—she never aspired to "keep up with the Joneses."

Nonetheless, she maintained cordial relations with Mrs. Andrew Carnegie and other society women, financially supporting their benefits and lending her name to their fundraising efforts—"Mrs. Walter G. Ladd" was frequently listed in the society column as a patroness, box holder, or "vice-chair" of a charitable event being held in New York City or Bar Harbor. She also maintained a constant friendship with John D. Rockefeller, Jr. who visited her frequently, especially in her later years. As her lawyer and friend Lawrence Morris recalled, whenever Rockefeller asked Kate to make a contribution to one of his many charities, she responded with a handsome donation and laughed, saying that "it was like taking coal to Newcastle, giving money to the Rockefellers" but since "this was where her fortune came from, she could never turn him down."[7]

Somewhat surprisingly, Kate was in good health overall in the years after her husband died, by which time Ludwig Kast was more sharply focused on his work with the Macy Foundation than on his patroness's day-to-day needs. He fully relinquished his role as Kate's medical doctor after suffering a heart attack in 1935. Having served as her physician for almost twenty years, Kast passed the reins to Dr. Andrew G. Foord, his wife Marie's brother-in-law. Foord might be perceived as a curious replacement since he did not conduct a private practice and lived a distance from Natirar; perhaps this choice signals that Kast wished to keep Kate's care "in the family." Foord operated the Nonkanahwa Sanitarium located near Kingston, New York, the hospital he had established in 1906. He served as both director and resident physician until his retirement in 1942. When he first examined Kate in February 1935, Dr. Foord said that he found her to be in much better health than most active people her age. He later commented that up until the end of her life she had no condition that required medical treatment other than the basic cold.[8] Kate's nurse companion Phyllis Temple (Ruby's replacement) agreed with Foord's assessment. She described her employer as an advocate of "preventive medicine." Kate had no chronic illness and took no regular medications—she followed a simple well-balanced diet and included some physical therapy and massage in her routine—all practices that are strikingly modern.

Foord and Temple's comments about the stability of Kate's health late in life are bolstered by those of Dr. Willard C. Rappleye. A

Foundation trustee, he assumed the presidency of the Macy
Foundation after Kast died in 1941. Rappleye brought a wealth of
experience to the organization as a distinguished physician, scholar,
and dean of the Columbia Medical School Faculty of Medicine, a
position he held from 1931-1958. He worked closely and compatibly
with Kate for a dozen years; as Foundation president he saw her every
two weeks, "always with the idea of telling her what was going on,
and she in turn showed the greatest interest in the various activities
and was particularly interested in some of the things we did for the
servicemen during the war."[9] He emphasized that Kate was extremely
active mentally and that she was "constantly alive" to problems in the
world. He valued her input—she was a woman who read a great deal
and made numerous suggestions regarding things that she was
interested in seeing the Foundation address.[10]

   Dr. Rappleye never viewed Kate as a sickly woman or an invalid,
and he considered her overall physical condition to be excellent. He
acknowledged that Kate chose to use a wheelchair or recline under the
general theory she would be a great deal better off if she did not
overdo things and use up her energy and described her lack of
mobility as a "functional disorder," which he called a "common
thing" that in no way interfered with her intellectual capacity.
However, it did cause her leg muscles to atrophy, making mobility
impracticable.[11] According to her attorney Lawrence Morris, Kate
expressed her belief that people would be better off if they spent
several days a month resting in bed—she thought that Americans
tended to exhaust themselves socially.[12]

   Much has been made of Kate's preference to stay off her feet as
well as her seclusion at Natirar after 1936, the basis for her being
called an invalid, but this depiction obscures both the vitality of her
mind and her deserved legacy as a significant advocate for health. It is
worth noting that Kate was not unique in promoting the need for rest.
Prominent individuals such as Henry Wadsworth Longfellow who
penned "Joy, temperance and repose, slam the door on the doctor's
nose" advocated for better living as an antidote for illness and by the
early twentieth century a "philosophy of rest," which sought to
counteract the hectic pace and "complexities" of life had become well
known. An influential proponent of rest as a cure for the "unrest" of
the day, Ella Adelia Fletcher, was a popular women's magazine

health and beauty writer and syndicated newspaper columnist. She also wrote health-related books. In her 1906 publication, *The Philosophy of Rest,* she said,

> We must teach men and women to combine activity with rest, to recognize that achievement is not always the result of struggle and strife; but that sometimes the greatest rewards, even of a purely worldly nature, are won by the leisurely expectant.[13]

Fletcher said that "hurry and worry" was a dangerous affliction that could be offset if one would "cultivate repose and a critical faculty of selection."[14] Her philosophy was adopted and promoted by the popular early twentieth century New Thought religious movement which Kate and Alice had explored. The movement emphasized health and healing at regular Sunday "services;" these were led by lay people, often women, and generally conducted in hotels or Masonic temples. Sermons addressed topics such as "The Science of Eternal Youth," "How to Better Your Position," and "Creating an Atmosphere of Health and Success." New Thought's spiritually healing talks attracted many people who were interested in the concept that would become known as "the power of positive thinking." It stands to reason that Kate and Alice were attracted to a philosophy that recognized the role of positive thinking in the quest for better health and it does not go unnoticed that during this period Kate's health was at its peak. In *Autumn Leaves from Maple Cottage,* her first book of inspiration for convalescents, we find further evidence of her belief in the importance of rest,

> Few people realize to what extent fatigue is responsible for ill-feelings and ill-thinking. Fatigue causes depression of body and spirit. It often poisons our thoughts and gives us distorted visions of life. Fatigue is not cured by excitement nor by play. The cure of fatigue is rest of body and mind accompanied by thoughts of peace and strength.[15]

In addition to reporting on her overall good health, the professionals who surrounded Kate in her final years emphasized her positivity; she was consistently remembered as a cheerful woman with an outlook that was optimistic and forward-looking, always planning ahead up until she became critically ill in the spring of 1945.[16] Miss Temple recalled Kate as a particularly happy woman, someone who was "young for her age...young in her ideas and thoughts." She "loved being with her girls...she loved to dress up and everything about her was young." Temple said that Kate had many visitors who came when invited, including young people.[17] Although Kate spent her time at Natirar after 1936, she was never reclusive. Regina O'Hara, a friend of Ruby Firlotte Meany remembered her visits to Natirar during the Christmas holidays in the 1930s. She was invited for lunch and O'Hara wrote, "While we did not eat with Mrs. Ladd...it was a beautiful sight to see the place glow with Christmas decorations." She said that it was, "an honor to have met such a wonderful woman. She was the essence of kindness to everyone."[18]

Nevertheless, as would be expected, the number of close friends and family members who regularly visited Kate had diminished to a trickle by the early 1940s—many of her contemporaries including Dora Van Wyck Schenk, Marie Ely Hill, and Lil Lemley McKeand had passed away. Everit's sons and daughter were focused on their own affairs. Val Jr.'s daughter Edith who had always maintained a close relationship with Kate was living with her mother Lydia and stepfather Ranieri Bourbon Del Monte Santa Maria, Prince di San Faustino in Rome. By the time she was able to leave Italy Kate had died.[19] Up until 1940, nephew Josiah Macy Willets was probably the family member most involved with Kate on a day-to-day basis; as a trustee of Walter's estate he worked closely with a staff of more than forty to carry Walter's meticulous management practices forward. Even after it was determined that Kate would no longer travel to Bar Harbor he insisted upon maintaining Eegonos in perfect condition in the event that Kate might wish to return. He supervised the extensive redecorating of the Natirar mansion house in accordance with Kate's wishes—furniture was reupholstered and paintings, carpets, and draperies were rehabilitated, and he saw to it that air conditioning was installed in her bedroom for her comfort. Willets oversaw both properties and consulted with his aunt regularly until he took his life in October 1940.

The decrease in visitors at Natirar further explains Kate's increased reliance upon key members of her staff, especially her chief nurse and estate supervisor. Her great niece believes that nurse companion Phyllis Temple, who was known to rule the roost, manipulated Kate during her final years.[20] Kate gave Miss Temple large monetary gifts in addition to her salary and the income that Kate provided through an earlier established trust fund. Kate also gave financial help to Temple's younger sister Gwyneth Philip who made frequent airplane trips from Toronto to New York between 1941 and 1945. Kate not only paid for some of these trips, she also added a codicil to her will to provide a $50,000 bequest for Mrs. Philip, an exorbitant sum considering the brief duration of their acquaintance.

Kate's other key employee and champion was estate superintendent Herbert William Tickner. He expressed concern about the way some staff members treated "Mrs. Ladd" and confided to his family that he thought that Miss Temple was out to "milk" their elderly employer for all she could.[21]

Kate enjoyed an easygoing relationship with Mr. Tickner who, like his predecessor Stanley Jones, was an Englishman. Tickner was a good fit at Natirar as he brought a wealth of experience to the post. He had been classically trained in England as a horticulturist and was a man with a passion for growing flowers; early in his career he had been employed nearby at Florham, the expansive Twombley estate and current home of Farleigh Dickinson University. According to a family story, he had applied for a job at Natirar about 1920 but Walter Ladd turned him down, telling the young gardener to come back once he was a married man. Tickner returned eighteen years later with his Danish-born wife and four children in tow. By that point, Walter had died. Nonetheless, the new superintendent upheld Walter's standard of perfection regarding every aspect of the Natirar estate management. He ensured that the extensive network of gravel and bluestone drives was groomed every Saturday by a crew of men who used herring bone rakes, and he saw to it that the lawns were lush and free of weeds. When the labor pool was reduced during World War II he brought in a herd of sheep to manicure the grass. Tickner insured that the large greenhouse and rose and cutting gardens and Maple Cottage vegetable garden were always in peak condition allowing flowers and food crops to thrive on the property; to Kate's delight fresh flowers were available to beautify her home in season. Tickner saw Kate regularly and called her "a wonderful woman." He was reportedly very protective of her and said that even though a nurse would try to take advantage of her (implicating Miss Temple) he felt that for the most part Mrs. Ladd was "in charge."[22] At some point Kate expressed her wish to have a pet, a small dog like Comus who could have provided comfort and companionship: She was told that a dog would cause too much excitement in the house. Kate had always been an animal lover so perhaps she shared her disappointment with Mr. Tickner. He began a tradition of visiting her with lambs, bunnies, and chicks in the spring, which may have coincided with Easter and her birthday. The nurses were temporarily overruled as Kate welcomed her small guests into the house; she was reportedly so happy to see the baby animals that she never cared if one of them "let loose" and made a mess.[23]

Beyond daily activities related to her home and staff and occasional visitors including Augusta Hope, Alice Vanderbilt Morris, and Emily Vanderbilt Hammond it was Kate's unceasing interest in the Macy Foundation and close relationship with Willard Rappleye that meant the most to her.

In 1943 Isaac Ogden Woodruff, a New York City doctor, took over her medical care. He had been an internist since 1904 and was known for his public health work; one of his specific interests was the eradication of tuberculosis. He joined the Macy Foundation board, serving as a trustee from 1943-1958. Sometime after 1945 he and Phyllis Temple married. The onset of Kate's final illness occurred in mid-1943. It was determined that she had developed breast cancer, but it was thought to be a sluggish and slow-growing form that could possibly linger for years. Woodruff never told Kate that she had cancer. Instead, he brought in a skin specialist who told her that she had eczema and prescribed a salve. It is likely that Phyllis Temple was the only member of her staff who knew the truth. For about one year Kate held her own and remained in "extraordinarily good condition." Woodruff believed that she might live for another ten or fifteen years. Nevertheless, the cancer advanced far more quickly than anticipated, and in 1945 at the age of eighty-two she suffered a serious attack of pneumonia. It was followed by a subsequent and fatal bout of the disease just a few weeks later.[24]

Kate passed away in the peaceful atmosphere of Natirar, her home of forty years, several hours before dawn on Monday, August 27, 1945. Dr. Rappleye had visited with her the day before. Since Dr. Woodruff was on holiday in Canada his assistant, Seward J. Handler, was overseeing her care; he had been out to see her two days before she died. It appears, however, that the junior doctor was not as well-informed about Kate's illness as he should have been. He incorrectly noted "Arterio Sclerosis, Heart Disease" as cause of death on her death certificate, a fact that Dr. Woodruff strenuously disputed. He stated his patient's death was a result of "a cancer which we had every reason to believe was penetrating her lung." Later Dr. Handler admitted that he had been in error.[25]

Kate's funeral service was held at the interdenominational Riverside Church in the Morningside Heights section of New York City on August 29, 1945. This was a significant venue due to her relationship with the two men who were most highly identified with the institution; John D. Rockefeller, Jr. who conceived and largely financed its construction and Harry Emerson Fosdick, Riverside's prominent liberal founding pastor. Both men were raised in the Baptist faith and as adults embraced the idea of a more modern ecumenical church that would welcome all who professed faith in Christ; in addition Riverside emphasized social outreach from its earliest days. Kate supported the ideological mission of Riverside and was also a contributor to the church through her lifelong loyalty to Rockefeller and personal admiration for Fosdick. Like millions of people worldwide, Kate was familiar with Mr. Fosdick through his weekly radio show "National Vespers Hour" which aired on NBC and short-wave radio from the late 1920s until 1946, bringing his skilled oratory and progressive beliefs into homes in seventeen countries. She thought so highly of the preacher, whom she never had met in person, that she invited him to join the board of the Josiah Macy Jr. Foundation. He served as a trustee from 1930, the year that Riverside held its first service, until 1961.[26]

More than seven decades after the event, we have a peek inside Riverside Church on August 29, 1945, through the recollection of one of Herbert Tickner's twin daughters, a self-described fifteen-year-old country bumpkin. Wearing her Sunday best, she and her family traveled from Natirar to the big city to pay their final respects to her father's employer: Tickner insisted on bringing his family to the funeral because he held Kate in such high regard. This was an astounding day in Miss Tickner's young life. She had never attended a funeral before, and her typical church experience centered on Sunday services at the charming and bucolic St. Luke's Episcopal Church located down the road from Natirar. She recalled that Riverside was like nothing she had ever encountered before—when the Neo-Gothic house of worship first opened detractors called it a monstrosity of enormous proportions. Nevertheless, the visitor from Peapack, New Jersey, was amazed by the sight of the building; it was undoubtedly the largest and tallest structure she had ever seen. The church easily held 2,500 people, and on that summer day the place was "packed." The young women's most abiding memory of the occasion was the remarkable profusion of flowers, "beds" of pink and white roses, on display throughout the church, a beautiful living reminder of Kate's loving and enduring spirit.[27]

Epilogue

AS WE HAVE LEARNED, Kate Macy Ladd's philosophy of health was uniquely ahead of its time. Relationships with her companion Alice Lemley as well as Drs. S. Weir Mitchell, Ludwig Kast, Helen Flanders Dunbar, and Willard Rappleye opened her eyes to new ways of thinking and led her to understand that health was far more than freedom from sickness. As her thinking evolved she progressed from being controlled by illness to becoming an ardent advocate for health.

A variety of experiences including an interest in positive thinking, a belief in the mind-body connection, and an understanding of the necessity of preventive medicine converged to help shape Kate's journey. It was through her exposure to spiritual alternatives and the reading of early twentieth century health books and articles that she became an early advocate of the power of positive thinking. This idea would eventually be popularized with the preaching and writing of Norman Vincent Peale who offered a remedy for spiritual, emotional, and physical malaise in his controversial 1952 best-seller *The Power of Positive Thinking*. In the twenty-first century we find that health advocates overwhelmingly address positive thinking as one of the necessary ingredients in the recipe for promoting physical and emotional health and forestalling disease.

Through Kate's "helpful talks" with health professionals she explored the notion of the mind-body connection—she first publicly advanced the belief that good health resided in the wholesome unity of mind and body when she established the Macy Foundation in 1930.[1] While the idea of a "wholesome unity of mind and body" was embraced by the Foundation and reflected in the work of Dr. Flanders Dunbar, this pioneering concept was ridiculed by the mainstream medical community for decades. It was not until the 1970s when documented evidence of the physiological link between mind and body was firmly established within the scientific community that the principle that one's mental state could influence susceptibility to disease became a more generally accepted view. Kate had experienced the joy of the unity of mind and body firsthand: When she was on firm ground emotionally her physical health was at its peak, as in her happy early years at Natirar and when she was fully engaged in the work of the Foundation toward the waning years of her life.[2]

The issue of preventive medicine was one that Kate championed in her own life. Based on her experience with her mother and sister who both succumbed to breast cancer in the 1890s, when she detected a tumor in her breast she knew that it was critical to act quickly—possibly saving her life. Recognition of the need for women to play a role in breast cancer prevention was articulated by the precursor to the American Cancer Society, established in New York City with her brother and his wife as founding members. In addition, Kate recommended topics for investigation by the Josiah Macy Jr. Foundation and supported the organization's research regarding some of the weightiest medical issues of the day. Close to home, in her work with the Visiting Nurse Association of New Jersey, she championed milk inspection to prevent the spread of illness in the community as well as vision and dental screening services for local schoolchildren. Kate's devotion to free convalescence for women in the gentle atmosphere of Maple Cottage is further evidence of her advanced thinking about health.

Much as Kate's philosophy and healthcare advocacy had a significant impact on ordinary people during her lifetime, her healthcare advocacy continues to resonate in the decades since her death. While her legacy is most visible through the continued vitality of the Josiah Macy Jr. Foundation, a closer look at the achievements of The Kate Macy Ladd Convalescent Home, created under the terms of Walter Ladd's will, is warranted.

By all accounts the mission of the convalescent home was highly ambitious—the fact that it was a stunning success speaks to both the Ladd's largesse and outstanding day-to-day management. Under the skillful administration of the Newark based Kate Macy Ladd Fund, the self-supporting convalescent home was tasked with providing a professionally planned and supervised medical and recreational program for women ages eighteen through sixty-nine.[3] The Kate

Macy Ladd Convalescent Home, probably the only entity ever named for Kate, has been called the standard bearer among similar institutions due to its conscientious and comprehensive medical care, dedicated staff, and the serene and welcoming outdoor environment of the Natirar estate which guests were encouraged to explore and enjoy. The facility was highly unique: It supplied free state-of-the-art care to more than 22,000 women referred by hundreds of doctors and hospitals between January 1949 and April 1983. As one hospital consultant said,

> Probably the most conspicuous example of convalescence par excellence is the Kate Macy Ladd Home in Far Hills, where through the most generous provision of its creator an extraordinarily complete array of diagnostic and therapeutic services is available in a setting probably unequalled for comfort and luxury and with an atmosphere conducive to the highest degree of guest morale.[4]

On January 17, 1949, the Home's first guest, Miss Etta Pfluger, was ushered through the front door of the mansion and into a handsome foyer. Gazing down to welcome her were Kate and Walter represented by newly rendered Albert Herter oil portraits, created from a composite of the Ladds' photographs. Kate appears as a young and attractive modern woman while Walter cuts a dashing figure—by contrast he is a slightly "older man" in his prime.

The striking portraits were not the only changes found in the Ladds' former home. The Tudor-style mansion was fully renovated to accommodate up to forty-nine women simultaneously on a year-round basis—more than twice the number served at Maple Cottage at a time—as well as a greatly expanded professional and service staff. While the number of women served remained fairly constant (on average about 625 women recuperated at the Home annually), the size and specialties of the staff increased over time to include physicians, nurses, aides, pharmacists, technicians, social workers, dieticians, chefs, physical and occupational therapists, recreation supervisors, housekeepers, laundresses, waitresses, and administrative staff. Many employees resided locally; noticeably absent were Phyllis Temple, Dr. Woodruff, and Kate's "in-house" staff. One exception was her superintendent, Herbert Tickner, who remained at his post and retained some of his building and grounds crew until he retired in

1952. His involvement eased the challenging transition from grand estate to a state-regulated medical facility.

By necessity, interior renovations altered the overall elegance of the main house. Despite this the most significant architectural elements of the home were spared. For example, the teak floors, carved oak and linenfold paneling, leaded windows, intricate plaster ceilings, and ornate fireplace mantels remained as originally designed by Guy Lowell. One month after Kate died the contents of her home—"Important Oil Paintings, Oriental Carpets, Furniture, Silver, Porcelains,"—were sold at public auction by Plaza Art Galleries, Inc. of East Fifty-Ninth Street.[5] The auction booklet called attention to 265 items and included everything from the previously advertised paintings and carpets to tables and chairs and even Walter's monogrammed linens and Turkish towels, leaving the house virtually empty and ready to remodel and redecorate. Essential to the conversion from mansion to medical facility was one regrettable modification—the removal of the mansion's grand staircase which was replaced with a service staircase and a modern institutional elevator that enabled guests to safely reach the upper two floors of the home. The bedrooms, which each accommodated two to four women, were located on the top floor; medical services were concentrated on the second floor, which also housed a small beauty shop where women enjoyed the psychological lift associated with a free hair styling upon arrival and at the end of their stay. The home's décor, which had been updated during the late 1930s, was completely modernized to reflect the times by L. Bamberger and Company of Newark; despite this turn toward contemporary design, guests were still expected to "dress" for dinner each evening.

Aspects of Kate's thinking about healthcare were in evidence at the home that bore her name. While necessary state-of-the-art medical and rehabilitative services were provided to the guests, and healthy and nourishing meals were offered, routine preventive health screenings were also made available. As medical director Dr. A.L Van Horn recognized, important strides had been made in cancer treatment for women. In a pamphlet distributed to guests he wrote that "the secret lies in its early recognition." To this end, the Home offered every woman the opportunity to schedule a Pap smear test while convalescing. Somewhat ironically, a small soda fountain and gift shop sold ice cream concoctions and sundries including cigarettes, a sign of the not yet changing times. It was also a casual gathering place, one of many spots inside the house and around the estate where women were encouraged to relax and enjoy each other's company. This ritual of women congregating companionably, developing friendships, and feeling more cheerful after suffering a physical or emotional setback harkens back to Kate's experience at the Lexington Sanitarium when she and her friends Marie and Nettie banded together to make the best of their situation.

For most women at the Kate Macy Ladd Convalescent Home, the emotional support they received was as beneficial as the expert care given. The warm and elegant environment, social activities, and interaction with compassionate staff members who were always available to "listen" hastened patient recovery. Guests universally sang the praises of what they called "The Kate Macy Ladd Home" and said that they received the royal treatment during their stay at Natirar. Few women could have imagined being cared for at this gracious place where dignity and compassion were dispensed to all. Furthermore, convalescing women had the opportunity to express personal concerns without shame or fear of retribution. As Winifred Skeat, director of Social Services, reported in 1982,

> In the many counseling interviews with patients, the main problem related to their families or home life, employment, financial concerns, or their adaptation to life as a single person. Emotional pressures were often aggravated by the impersonal, often intimidating environment of the modern hospital and the scientific technological changes. The Home offered the opportunity for them to freely verbalize anxieties, a chance to regain their self-sufficiency and return home with a link to community agencies if needed.[6]

With its emphasis on medical, recreational, and counseling services the convalescent home on the magnificent Ladd estate offered women a new lease on life. On their day of departure each guest received a fresh corsage to wear out into the world. The corsages were created with flowers from the estate's cutting garden or greenhouse, a lovely gesture that undoubtedly would have pleased Kate a great deal. It is no wonder that many women were reluctant to take leave of this place of gentle respite, a place that guests called "fairyland."

Between 1949 and 1983, the Home received hundreds of unsolicited comments from doctors, guests, and family members. Busy physicians found the time to express their appreciation for a patient's placement at the Home, "Thank you so much for the exquisite care given Mrs. Y. You are doing a magnificent job. S. D. M.D." Similarly, messages from guests exemplified the positive impact of their stay. In the words of one woman, "To have lived with the traditions left by Mr. and Mrs. Ladd and to be surrounded with so much of the beauty which they created has been a rare experience. I have come home not only much stronger but with a renewed spirit and a serenity which I could not have achieved alone. E. Q."

Another convalescent wrote, "The friendly and gracious atmosphere made me truly feel like a guest and not a convalescent; and your concern with our psychological as well as physical needs made a deep and lasting impression upon me. R. Y." Even grateful husbands sent notes of thanks, "As you know Mrs. J. has had a pretty rough time most of her life and she was pretty well down mentally at the time she went to Kate Macy Ladd. Since her return she has had an entirely new outlook on life and is her old happy self. Both she and I attribute this change to the wonderful kindness shown during her stay at Kate Macy Ladd. Mr. A. J."

To universal disappointment, as Walter Ladd's will specified, the Kate Macy Ladd Convalescent Home closed on May 21, 1983, fifty years after his death. Marketing to sell the mansion and the estate's remaining 490 acres had been set in motion the previous year. Natirar was ultimately sold to King Hassan II of Morocco for $7.5 million, breaking all records for home sales in the state of New Jersey, the previous highest sale price having been paid by automaker John DeLorean and his wife when they purchased a mansion with similar acreage in Bedminster for $3.5 million in 1981. Before the king began the process of converting the mansion from a convalescent home to what was expected to be a home fit for royalty the mansion house was emptied. Ten truckloads of furniture were transported to Hampton Institute a beneficiary of Walter's will; this made it possible for the school to furnish its new forty-five bed infirmity. Ladd descendants had the opportunity to purchase items that held special meaning. Monies realized from the sale of Natirar and an auction of contents of the mansion, as well as funds held in trust since the time of Walter's death were divided equally among five institutions that the Ladds supported during their lifetime. They included Berry School, Hampton Institute, Johns Hopkins Hospital, New York University Medical School, and Tuskegee Institute.[7]

King Hassan II officially took possession of Kate and Walter's former home on May 31, 1983. It was reported that he planned to use Natirar as his personal residence when visiting the United States. His name quickly became synonymous with the estate. It was as if all traces of Kate and Walter Ladd had suddenly evaporated. A new generation of well-heeled residents were intrigued by the exotic specter of a monarch in their midst and may have anticipated that his presence among them would further elevate the panache of their community. In June 1983 the King was welcomed into the neighborhood at a tony dinner-dance, which was meant to raise funds for the local PBS station. The event was held at a nearby estate that had been transformed into a "Moroccan Fantasy" for the occasion. A camel wandered about the grounds, and a tented marketplace, authentic Moroccan band, and veiled belly dancer brought the theme to life; guests included local politicians and luminaries such as Malcolm S. Forbes and Doris Duke. The King, however, was not on hand to meet his new neighbors; he sent a small delegation of his countrymen to represent him.[8] As things turned out, the King's affluent neighbors did not derive much benefit from his tenure in New Jersey. He never completed the extensive renovations that would have transformed the mansion house into a royal residence nor did he ever occupy the mansion house. Upon his death in 1999, his son King Mohammed VI inherited the estate. In March 2003, Somerset County purchased Natirar from the government of Morocco for $22 million.

Incredibly, an entire decade has passed since the Sunday when I first discovered the Somerset County Park that was once the estate of Kate Macy and Walter Ladd and felt inspired to learn more about the wealthy woman who created Maple Cottage. Unexpectedly the process of *Finding Kate* spawned a journey that I never imagined. As I quickly realized in order to truly find Kate, I needed access to primary document which necessitated finding individuals who had some type of relationship with her. My quest took me from New England, the Mid-Atlantic, and California to County Cork, Ireland. I met with many of Kate's descendants and the descendants of her former employees. Wherever I traveled I was warmly welcomed and graciously entertained. When it was time to say farewell, I emerged with fresh insights about Kate, and armed with documents, photographs, memorabilia, and gifts. Kate's essence literally surrounds me—her engagement quilt is one of my most beloved possessions; family photographs grace my home. Through regular conversations and correspondence my trove of information grew, enriching my research and making it more possible to tell Kate's story. I have also had the privilege of exploring the interiors of both of Kate's homes; Eegonos (currently called East of Eden) on the waterfront in Bar Harbor and Natirar. It was wonderful to see that Eegonos has been painstakingly restored to its original glory while Natirar is being reborn as a hospitality destination.

I return to the county park known as Natirar often. Over the years hiking there has soothed my soul and connected me to Kate's loving spirit. It is a particular thrill to know that Natirar has become one of Somerset County's best loved parks—on any given day children frolic on the massive lawn, kites and Frisbees catch the breeze, and dogs of every breed scamper in the fresh air. It is a place of peace and serenity. I am quite certain that the knowledge of all this would make Kate's kind heart sing with joy.

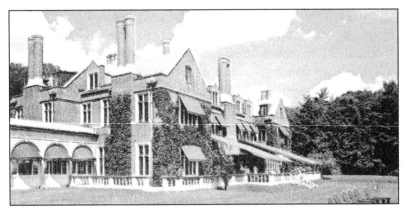

Terrace view of the Kate Macy Ladd Convalescent Home *(From an undated brochure produced by the Kate Macy Ladd Fund, Newark, NJ)*

Acknowledgments

I OWE A TREMENDOUS DEBT OF GRATITUDE to the many individuals who helped to make *Finding Kate* a reality. Above all I am indebted to my patient and supportive husband; his superior driving skills, love of travel, and good company enhanced the pleasure of my journey. I also offer my deepest thanks to my uncle Leonard Mellman, whose encouragement and love of history fueled my passion every step of the way. I would also like to thank my mother Sharlyn Weitz who nurtured my love of reading, which set me on this path. I am especially grateful to my friend and colleague W. Barry Thomson. His generous research assistance and our extensive and lively conversations about Kate and her milieu make this a far better book. My dear friend, foremost costume and textile historian Edward Maeder always cheered me on and shared his exemplary knowledge of quilts and fashion. It was always enlightening to discuss Kate and examine the lives of women of her era with Kathy Thurber. Special love and hugs go out to my closest friends and family members for putting up with my "Kate obsession" for so many years.

Through the intricate web of my research, personal introductions, and sometimes pure serendipity, I managed to find members of Kate's family as well as descendants of her employees. It would have been impossible to bring Kate's story to life without their involvement.

Kate's delightful great niece Edith Macy Shoenborn shared many charming stories and memories of her beloved aunt. Our visits were a special treat filled with good food and helpful conversation. Edith presented me with the unexpected gift of Kate's engagement quilt, knowing that it would hold special meaning for me, and she also introduced me to her cousins Archer and Janet Macy, faithful stewards of a collection of Macy family documents spanning the past two centuries. They generously made their family archives—hundreds of letters, diaries, photographs, and ephemera—available to me. Melanie Willets Sharp-Bolster, a great granddaughter of Kate's sister

Mae, entertained me at her home in County Cork, Ireland, where we poured over letters, photographs, and linens. Our discussions, boosted by Mel's delicious brown bread and cups of fortifying tea, amplified my understanding of the Willets branch of Kate's family. Deborah Macy, a distant cousin, introduced me to the wonders of the *Macy Genealogy,* which had been passed on to her through her father's branch of the family. I was also fortunate to discover descendants on Walter Ladd's side of the family. Frances Ladd Hundt, Rebe and Jim's great-granddaughter, has been a steady presence throughout my years of research and writing. Her warmth and intelligent insights have nurtured me endlessly.

Relatives of Kate's key employees have also provided me with their perceptions and a unique array of primary sources. Diane Conrad, Alice Lemley's great niece, and her husband offered me hospitality at their home as I perused Alice's guest book, scrapbooks, jewelry, and photographs surrounded by her original Maine bungalow furnishings. After a lengthy search I met Scott Fisher, Ruby's beloved grandson who grew up hearing about "Mrs. Ladd's" kindness and largesse; he filled in poignant details about Kate's relationship with her favorite nurse. Edith Tickner Silver shared her memories of Kate's funeral as well as photos and anecdotes from her father William H. Tickner's tenure as Natirar superintendent. Without question my biggest surprise while "finding Kate" came as I was tracking down Maple Cottage's first superintendent H. Estelle Dudley. I discovered that she was the great-great aunt of my college roommate Millicent Dudley Lake: Implausibly I spent the summer of 1976 in the village where Estelle was born, living a stone's throw away from her house on Main Street. I walked daily past the cemetery where she was laid to rest. Before I contacted her, my friend was not aware of Estelle and was unconvinced that there was a Dudley family connection to Kate. Then she discovered "Aunt Stella's" ledger book buried in a barrel of family memorabilia, which led us to work together to stitch Estelle's piece of Kate's story.

I had the unique opportunity to explore both of Kate's homes, visiting in her New Jersey mansion with a top to bottom tour, thanks to Thomas Boccino, Principal Planner, Land Acquisition, Somerset County Engineering Division. The magic of the meticulously restored Eegonos (now called East of Eden) was shared with me through the gracious hospitality of the late William B. Ruger, Jr. and Michael Hallet, who has tended the villa with the upmost care for more than forty years.

My research efforts were further enhanced through the assistance of several institutions and individuals. While roaming through the storage area at the Visiting Nurse Association of Somerset Hills headquarters in Basking Ridge, New Jersey I discovered meeting record books from Kate's era of association involvement. I received much helpful information including copies of personal letters pertaining to Kate and Berry College from Michael O'Malley and staff at Berry College Archives in Rome, Georgia. Mary B. Hotaling, Saranac Lake based biographer of Edward L. Trudeau, provided the important and revealing Trudeau-Ladd correspondence while the staff at the Josiah Macy Jr. Foundation welcomed me to their archives in New York City. Visits to the archives at the College of Physicians in Philadelphia unveiled the world of Victorian doctors and their medical practices and research at the Westchester County Archives in Elmsford, New York provided additional background material about Kate's immediate family.

It has been a pleasure to work with my supportive and resolute publisher Karen Hodges Miller of Open Door Publications and her staff. Karen was always available to offer encouragement and sleuth out the issues that accompany any manuscript, especially one with endless endnotes. She and proofreader Vivian Fransen provided thoughtful comments and editing expertise, and *Finding Kate* has been graced by the timeless artistry of designer Eric Labacz—the icing on the cake!

Last, but not least, I am indebted to my sons, Ben and Sam, who have unknowingly inspired me since they were born. It is my deepest wish that all of their future journeys will be filled with great excitement and the joy of discovery.

Endnotes

Chapter 2

[1] Henry R. Stiles, *History of the City of Brooklyn, N.Y. including the Old Town and Village of Brooklyn, the Town of Bushwick, and the Village and City of Williamsburgh, Volume* II, (Brooklyn: Published by Subscription, 1869), pp. 125-127.

[2] Edward Pessen, *Riches, Class, and Power: America Before the Civil War*, (New Brunswick and London: Transaction Publishers, 2009), pp. 179-180.

Chapter 3

[1] Silvanus J. Macy, *Genealogy of the Macy Family from 1635-1868*, (Albany: Joel Munshall, 1868), pp. 13-14.

[2] Ibid, p. 14.

[3] Ibid, p. 22.

[4] Ibid.

[5] Based on photographs and interview with Melanie Willets Campbell Sharp-Bolster, Kate's great-great niece, May 2016, Kanturk, Ireland.

[6] Ibid, p. 183.

[7] Silvanus J. Macy, p. 184.

[8] Ibid.

[9] As quoted in Allan Nevins, *The Evening Post: A Century of Journalism*, (New York: Boni and Liveright, 1922), p. 64.

Chapter 4

[1] Eleanor Leggett, Undated Essay.

Chapter 5

[1] From a letter written by Josiah Macy Jr. to Mary Macy Kingsland, April 1876. This was probably the last time that Josiah and Carrie traveled alone together before his death six months later.

[2] H. Larry Ingle, *Quakers in Conflict, The Hicksite Reformation*, (Wallingford, PA: Pendle Hill Press, 1998), p. 19.

[3] William Penn's Advice to His Children, Philadelphia Friends Council on Education, p. 15.

[4] J. William Frost, "As the Twig is Bent: Quaker Ideas of Childhood," *Quaker History* 60, #2, (1971) and Walter Homan, *Children and Quakerism: A Study of the Place of Children in the Theory and Practice of the Society of Friends, Commonly Called Quakers*, (Berkeley: Gillick Press, 1939), p. 9.

[5] Silvanus J. Macy, p. 24.

6 From a letter written by William M. Kingsland to William and Eliza Macy, August 24, 1875.

7 From a letter written by William H. Macy to Mary and William Kingsland, December 3, 1865.

Chapter 6

1 From a letter written by Josiah Macy Jr. to Mary Macy Kingsland, January 1, 1865.

2 *The Gentleman's Companion of 1870: New York City,* author and publisher unknown.

3 *The New York Times,* "Dens of Iniquity," January 26, 2011.

Chapter 7

1 *The Cleveland Leader*, January 19, 1870.

2 As related by Kate's nephew Noel Macy to Fred Irwin, 1975.

3 *The New York Times*, March 6, 1874.

4 From an unpublished biography of V.E. Macy by William C. Wright, Westchester County Archives Series: 187, V. Everit Macy Papers, 1900-1977.

5 From a letter written by William M. Kingsland to Josiah Macy Jr., March 24, 1876.

6 From a letter written by Josiah Macy Jr. to Mary and William Kingsland, April 10, 1876.

7 *The New York Times,* October 7, 1876.

8 For further detail about the Exposition see James D. McCabe, *The Illustrated History of the Centennial Exhibition,* (Philadelphia: National Publishing Company, 1876).

Chapter 8

1 Kate Macy Ladd, (KML), *The Story of My Life,* (Portland, ME: Mosher Press, 1930), p. 9.

2 Ibid.

3 From an undated letter (circa October 7, 1876) from Caroline Everit Macy to her children.

4 *The New York Times*, October 6, 1876.

5 From a letter written by William M. Kingsland to William and Eliza Macy, April 20, 1877.

6 Ibid, February 9, 1877.

7 Ibid, April 20, 1877.

8 Ibid, January 27, 1877.

9 Ibid, April 28, 1877.

10 W.H. Rideing, "Hospital Life in New York," *Harper's New Monthly Magazine*, Volume 57, Issue 338, (July 1878).

[11] Benson J. Lossing, *History of New York City: Embracing An Outline Sketch of Events From 1630 to 1830 And A Full Account of Its Development From 1830 to 1884*, (New York: A.S. Barnes and Co., 1884), p. 113.
[12] KML, pp. 11-12.
[13] Samuel Bowles, *The Switzerland of America, A Summer Vacation In the Mountains of Colorado*, (Springfield, MA: Samuel Bowles and Company, 1869).

Chapter 9
[1] KML, p. 16.
[2] Ibid., pp. 14-16.
[3] Raymond B. Fosdick, *John D. Rockefeller, Jr.: A Portrait*, (New York: Harper and Brothers, 1956), p. 35.
[4] *Richfield Springs Mercury,* Vol. 16, No. 4, July 30, 1881.
[5] Karl A. Cherry, "Devonport A Century Ago," *Western Morning News*, 1911.
[6] Ibid.
[7] *Genealogy of the Beach Family of Connecticut with Portions of the Genealogies of the Allied Families of Demmond, Walker, Gooding and Carpenter*, compiled by Charles C. McClaughry; c. 1905.
[8] Rebecca Donaldson Beach and Rebecca Donaldson Gibbons, *The Reverend John Beach and His Descendants*, (New Haven: The Tuttle, Morehouse and Taylor Press, 1898), p. 132.
[9] Ibid, pp. 86-120.
[10] Ibid, p. 160.
[11] William Cothren, *History of Ancient Woodbury, Connecticut*, (Waterbury, CT: Bronson Brothers, 1854), pp. 727-731.
[12] Christopher Grasso, *A Speaking Aristocracy: Transforming Public Discourse in Eighteenth-Century Connecticut*, (Chapel Hill and London: University of North Carolina Press, 1999), pp. 420-21.
[13] Ibid.
[14] Charles S. Brigham, "Bibliography of American Newspapers, 1620-1820," Proceedings of the Antiquarian Society, New Series, Vol. 27, April 11, 1917-October 17, 1917, (Worcester, MA: The Davis Press, 1917), p. 452.
[15] From a conversation with Ladd descendent F. Hundt, 2012.
[16] Excerpted from St. Andrew's Society of New York Constitution, City of New York, on the Thirteenth Day of November 1794.
[17] William M. MacBean, *Biographical Register of Saint Andrew's Society of the State of New York, Vol. 4*, (Printed for the Society), pp. 125-126.
[18] Westchester County, NY Deed, Liber #105, pp. 48-55, November 21, 1843.
[19] Throggs Neck was part of Westchester County until 1898, at which time it was incorporated into New York City.

Chapter 10
[1] KML, p. 17.
[2] Ibid, p. 18.
[3] From a conversation with Macy descendent Deborah Macy, 2008.
[4] KML, p. 18.
[5] Ibid.
[6] Ibid.
[7] Ibid, pp. 18-19.
[8] Ibid, p. 17.
[9] Ibid, p. 19.
[10] Ibid, p. 20.
[11] Ibid, pp. 21-22.
[12] Ibid, pp. 22-23.

Chapter 11
[1] Cindy Brick, *Crazy Quilts*, (St. Paul: Voyageur Press, 2008), pp. 33-34.
[2] As quoted in Lydia Bodman Vaderbergh and Earle G. Shettleworth, Jr. *Opulence to Ashes: Bar Harbor's Gilded Century, 1850-1950*, (Camden, ME: Down East Books, 2009), p. 45.
[3] Ibid, p. 96 and G.W. Helfrich and Gladys O'Neill, *Lost Bar Harbor,* (Camden, ME: Down East Books, 1982), p. 6.
[4] *Bar Harbor Times*, May 1900.
[5] As quoted in Elizabeth Flock, "Queen Victoria Was the First to Get Married in White," *The Washington Post*, April 29, 2011.
[6] Florence Hartley, *The Ladies Book of* Etiquette *and Manual of Politeness*, (New York: Lee, Shepard and Dillingham, 1872), p. 259.
[7] KML, p. 24.
[8] *Brooklyn Daily Eagle*, December 7, 1883, p. 3.

Chapter 12
[1] KML, p. 25.
[2] Henry Jellet, *Manual of Midwifery for Students and Practitioners*, (New York: William Wood and Co., 1905), pp. 567-569.
[3] Thomas T. Gaillard, *Abortion and Its Treatment From the Stand-Point of Practical Experience*, (New York: D. Appleton and Co., 1890), pp. 19-20.
[4] Thomas Trotter, *View of the Nervous Temperament; Being a Practical Inquiry into the Increasing Prevalence, Prevention, and Treatment of Those Diseases Commonly Called Nervous, Bilious, Stomach, Liver Complaints, Indigestion, Low-Spirits, Gout, Etc.,* (Troy, NY: Wright, Goodenow and Stockwell, 1897), pp. 41 and 51.
[5] KML, p. 26.
[6] Ibid.
[7] "The Canadian Journal of Medical Science," Vol. 6, 1881, p.93.

[8] See Theodore Gaillard Thomas, *A Practical Treatise on the Diseases of Women*, (Philadelphia: Henry C. Lea, 1869).

[9] Ibid, p. 6.

[10] Margaret Marsh and Wanda Ronner, *The Empty Cradle, Infertility in America from Colonial Times to the Present*, (Baltimore: The Johns Hopkins Press, 1996), pp. 50-52.

[11] Ibid, pp. 82-86.

[12] KML, p. 28.

[13] Ibid.

[14] Ronald C. White, *American Ulysses: A Life of Ulysses S. Grant*, (New York, NY: Random House, 2016), pp. 627-629.

[15] Geoffrey C. Ward, *A Disposition to be Rich, Ferdinand Ward, the Greatest Swindler of the Gilded Age*, (New York: Vintage Books, 2013), p. 197.

Chapter 13

[1] Robert A. M. Stern, Thomas Mellins and David Fishman, *New York 1880: Architecture and Urbanism in the Gilded Age*, (New York; Monacelli Press, 1999), p. 552.

Chapter 14

[1] *The New York Tribune*, January 24, 1886.

[2] From a letter dated January 27, 1886, written by Howard Willets to Mary Macy Kingsland. It is interesting to note that Howard spells his wife's name "May" whereas she and the family spell it "Mae."

[3] KML, p. 30.

[4] Ibid, pp. 30-31.

[5] From a letter dated February 18, 1888, written by Anna Paret to Kate Macy Ladd and M.E.F. Friends.

[6] KML, p. 33.

[7] Ibid.

[8] William Mill Butler, *The Whist Reference Book*, (Philadelphia: John C. Yorston Co., 1898), p. 94.

[9] Ibid, p. 95.

Chapter 15

[1] KML, p. 35.

[2] Ibid.

Chapter 16

[1] KML, p. 42.

[2] Dr. Fordyce Barker had previously studied and labeled the preponderance of nervous disease associated with the northeastern United States "nervous

asthenia." Beard, Barker, and alienist Van Deusen had been similarly influenced by the work of Austin Flint. His 1866 medical textbook included a section titled "Nervous Asthenia." David G. Schuster, "Neurasthenic Nation: The Medicalization of Modernity in the United States, 1869-1920," Dissertation, University of California, Santa Barbara, 2006, pp. 2, 50, and 73.

[3] George Miller Beard, *A Practical Treatise on Nervous Exhaustion (neurasthenia); Its Symptoms, Nature, Sequences, Treatment,* (New York: Wood, 1880).

[4] David G. Schuster, "Neurasthenic Nation: The Medicalization of Modernity in the United Sates, 1869-1920," Dissertation, University of California, Santa Barbara, 2006, p. 2.

[5] Ibid, p. 71. For an in-depth discussion of the evolution of the medical shaping of psychosomatic symptoms see Edward Shorter, *From Paralysis To Fatigue: A History of Psychosomatic Illness in the Modern Era*, (New York: The Free Press, 1992), pp. 5-25.

[6] Anne Stiles, "The Rest Cure, 1873-1925," BRANCH: Britain, Representation and Nineteenth-Century History. Dino Franco Felluga, Ed., Extension of Romanticism and Victorianism on the Net.Web. 2016.

[7] Tom Lutz, *American Nervousness, 1903, An Anecdotal History,* (Ithaca, NY: Cornell University Press 1991), pp. 2-3 and Francis G. Gosling, *Before Freud: Neurasthenia and the American Medical Community, 1870-1910,* (Urbana, IL: University of Illinois Press, 1987), p. xi.

[8] Nancy Cervetti, "S. Weir Mitchell: The Early Years, APS Bulletin," March/April 2003, p. 7.

[9] Ibid, p. 8.

[10] Ibid, p. 7.

[11] Nancy Cervetti, *S. Weir Mitchell, 1829-1914: Philadelphia's Literary Physician,* (University Park, PA: The Pennsylvania State University Press, 2012), pp. 105-108.

[12] S. Weir Mitchell, *Fat and Blood: An Essay on Certain Forms of Neurasthenia and Hysteria,* (London and Philadelphia: J.B. Lippincott Company 8th Edition, 1911), pp. 1 and 15.

[13] Ibid, p. 22.

[14] KML, p. 46.

Chapter 17
[1] KML, p. 47.
[2] Ibid, p. 48.
[3] S. Weir Mitchell, *Fat and Blood,* p. 5.
[4] Ibid, pp. 49-50.

Chapter 18
[1] Edward Wakefield, "Nervousness: The National Disease of America," *McClure's Magazine*, Vol. II, December 1893, S.S. McClure Limited, N.Y. and London, p. 302.
[2] Ruth J. Abram, Ed., *Send Us A Lady Physician: Women Doctors in America 1835-1920*, (New York, NY: W.W. Norton & Co., Inc., 1985), pp. 96-98.
[3] Westchester County Records, Liber #1334, p. 211.

Chapter 19
[1] KML,pp. 52-53.
[2] Ibid, p. 53.
[3] Henry Fry, *The History of North American Steam Navigation,* (London: Samson, Low, Marston and Co., 1896), pp. 175-176.
[4] The events of February 1892 were reconstructed from assorted contemporaneous columns, which appeared in *The New York Times* during the first and second weeks of February 1892 as well as August 8, 1892.

Chapter 20
[1] *The Century Illustrated Monthly Magazine, Vol. XXXIII, No. 5* (New York: The Century Co., March, 1887), p. 40.
[2] John W. Rae, *Morristown, A Military Headquarters of the American Revolution,* (Charleston, SC, Chicago, Portsmouth, NH and San Francisco: Arcadia Publishing 2002), p. 85.

Chapter 21
[1] *The Los Angeles Times,* July 10, 1897.
[2] Ibid, January 1, 1898.
[3] Ibid, September 18, 1898.

Chapter 22
[1] *The Los Angeles Times,* April 4, 1899, p. 13.
[2] Philip L. Gallos, *Cure Cottages of Saranac Lake*, (Historic Saranac Lake, Saranac Lake, NY 1985), p. 16.
[3] *Nursing History Review,* 19: 2011, pp. 29-52.
[4] This marked the beginning of a forty year period of living in the Adirondacks.
[5] See also Edward Livingston Trudeau, M.D., *An Autobiography,* (Garden City, NY: Doubleday, Doran & Co., 1936).
[6] Trudeau also treated a number of affluent and distinguished patients including financial supporter George Campbell Cooper and author Robert Louis Stevenson who worked and convalesced at Saranac Lake for six months between 1887 and 1888.
[7] *British Journal of Tuberculosis,* Vol. 2, Issue 4, October 1908, p. 279.

[8] The fair was held at Paul Smith's for many years, and the proceeds provided considerable funding for the sanitarium. Kate and her mother donated items for the sale, and in a letter that Walter wrote to Mrs. Elizabeth Milbank in August, 1899 he mentioned that Kate was sending several items to be sold at the annual fundraising event.

[9] Mary B. Hotaling, *A Rare Romance in Medicine: The Life and Legacy of Edward Livingston Trudeau*, (Saranac Lake, NY: Historic Saranac Lake, 2016), pp. 74-75.

[10] It was customary to refer to such cottages by the name of the donor. Ladd Cottage stands on its original plot of land and is listed on the National Register of Historic Places.

[11] From a letter written by Walter G. Ladd to Edward L. Trudeau, August 15, 1899.

[12] From a letter written by Walter G. Ladd to the Trustees of the Adirondack Cottage Sanitarium, August 24, 1899.

[13] Coulter's work at the A.C.S. paved the way for a lucrative career in the region. See Mary B. Hotaling, "W.L. Coulter, Architect," *Adirondack Architectural Heritage Newsletter,* Vol. 4, Number 2, December 1995.

[14] Based on an interview with Michele Tucker, Curator Adirondack Research Center, Saranac Lake, NY 2017. For further detail about the life and work of E.L. Trudeau see Mary B. Hotaling, A *Rare Romance in Medicine: The Life and Legacy of Edward Livingston Trudeau*, (Saranac Lake, NY: Historic Saranac Lake, 2016).

[15] From a letter written by C.R. Armstrong to Dr. E.R. Baldwin, May 1, 1928, Saranac Institute Library.

Chapter 23

[1] Ulto is an abbreviation for the Latin ultimo meaning "last month" and was in common use during the eighteenth and nineteenth centuries.

[2] From a letter written by Walter G. Ladd to Dr. E.L. Trudeau, June 18, 1900.

[3] KML, p. 67.

[4] In 1904, several years after the Curies had discovered and isolated radium, Abbe brought a supply of the element to the United States from their laboratory in Paris for use in his surgical practice. For more about Robert Abbe se, "Robert Abbe: The Life and Times of a 19th Century Surgeon," Steven G. Friedman *Journal of Vascular Surgery*, 2017:66: pp. 1290-1292.

[5] *Medical Record,* Vol. 57. George F. Shrady, Ed., (New York: Wm. Wood and Co., 1900).

[6] Ellen Leopold, *A Darker Ribbon: Breast Cancer, Women and Their Doctors in the Twentieth Century,* (Boston: Beacon Press, 1999), p. 37.

[7] Ibid, pp. 37 and 49.

[8] James S. Olson*, Bathsheba's Breast: Women, Cancer and History*, (Baltimore and London: The Johns Hopkins University Press, 2002), p. 33.

[9] Ibid, p. 40.

[10] Ibid, pp. 40-44.

[11] From a memorandum written by Mrs. Ladd's personal secretary Phoebe Edgar circa 1949.

[12] *The New York Times*, July 1, 1900.

[13] Ibid. McMillan built Elsinore in 1893-94. He subsequently leased the house to the Ladds for a few years and then sold it to Susan Whitney Dimock, a leader in Bar Harbor's social and civic affairs and a Bar Harbor mainstay for more than sixty years.

[14] *The New York Times,* August 12, 1900.

Chapter 24

[1] KML, pp. 68-69.

[2] Ibid, pp. vi and 113.

[3] Ibid, p. 68.

[4] Ibid, p. 70.

[5] Adding insult to injury, details of the will appeared in local newspapers.

[6] Edgar Memorandum. The Ladds' financial agreement remained in effect until December 31, 1929. Upon termination, Walter received a final payment of $829,501.94, the equivalent of roughly twelve million dollars in 2016 dollars. During the final quarter of 1929, Kate was dictating her memoir to her secretary and finalizing plans to provide a multi-million dollar gift to create a foundation in memory of her father. Although the nation was reeling from the effects of Black Friday, the stock market crash of 1929 did not have an affect on her finances.

[7] Edgar Memorandum.

[8] The Ladds also purchased an additional 150 acres from William Stone Post, 95 acres from Alletta and John DeBaun, and 75 acres from Evander H. Schley.

[9] "Natirar: A Study of the Estate of the King of Morocco," The Somerset County Park Commission, The Natirar Association, Inc., The RBA Group and the Upper Raritan Watershed Association, 2002. The history section was written by W. Barry Thomson.

[10] Based on the research of W. Barry Thomson, "The Farm and Barns of Sunnybranch Farm/Natirar," 2008.

[11] KML, p. 93.

[12] Ibid, pp. 69-72.

[13] According to Vivienne Peterson of the Pomeranian Project, quite a few Poms of this era were named after literary characters. Comus was featured in Greek mythology and a work of Milton.

[14] *The New York Times*, January 8, 1911.

[15] Ibid.

Chapter 25

[1] Florence Nightingale, *Notes on Hospitals,* (London: Longman, Green, Longman, Roberts and Green, 1863), p. 107.

[2] Edythe Lane Van Doren was related to one of the settlers of the Nevius-Lane tract, which formed the nucleus of the Natirar estate. See William A. and Amanda R. Schleicher, *Images of America: Bedminster*, (Charleston, SC: Arcadia Publishing), 1998.

[3] Blockley Hospital was renamed the Philadelphia General Hospital in 1902. The P.G.H. School of Nursing was a mainstay of nursing education for ninety years. The school's final class graduated in the spring of 1977. See Stephanie A. Stachniewicz and Jean K. Axelrod, *The Double Frill: The History of the Philadelphia General Hospital School of Nursing*, (Philadelphia: George F. Stickley Co., 1978).

[4] As noted in the *Hamilton Spectator*, January 15, 1912, p. 14, in honor of the Lemley-McKeand nuptials, Mrs. Beardmore hosted a "very large tea." Hundreds of guests, including the bride's sister, Alice Lemley, lingered well after the party was to end. The groom, David Livingstone McKeand, became a well-known Canadian Arctic explorer.

[5] From the lecture notes of Alice Lemley, March 15, 1888, Blockley Hospital (Bates Nursing Archives, University of Pennsylvania, MC 53).

[6] *The Free Press*, November 13, 1903.

[7] From a letter written by Estelle Dudley to Jeanie Dudley Murphy, February 3, 1907.

[8] *The Bernardsville News,* June 4, 1909.

[9] *The American Journal of Nursing*, Vol. 9, No. 10, July 1909, p. 759.

[10] KML, p. 71.

[11] From a typed memo from Maple Cottage written by Miss H. Estelle Dudley, Supt. Macy Family Archives.

[12] KML, p. 81.

[13] *Autumn Leaves From Maple Cottage* (Portland, ME, The Mosher Press, 1919) and *Spring Blossoms From Maple Cottage* (Portland, ME, The Mosher Press, 1928). Although Kate compiled and financed the printing of the volumes, she did so anonymously, as was her way.

[14] From a postcard written by Josephine Burroughs to her friend Harrie Young. Miss Burroughs was a self-supporting woman who made her living as a writer. She convalesced at Maple Cottage between September 14 and 28, 1938.

Chapter 26
[1] Carrie wanted her building to teach the manual arts, a pet interest of her son Everit. Initially, the building was called the Macy Manual Arts Building, later Macy Hall. See Andrew S. Dolkart, *Morningside Heights, A History of Its Architecture and Development,* (New York, NY: Columbia University Press, 1998), pp. 227-230.

[2] Ibid, p. 243.

[3] This was probably a coincidence. Even though Kahn maintained a residence in Morristown, "Cedar Court," for two decades, it does not appear that the Ladds and the Kahns were socially friendly.

[4] KML, p. 84. C. B. Mitchell and his wife Mildred Matthews Mitchell lived nearby on the Bernardsville Mountain at "Pennwood." Mrs. Mitchell was a doctor's daughter and a leading member of the local Visiting Nurse Association, which is where she and Kate became acquainted. The architect Chester Aldrich and his sister Amy were old Macy family friends. Chester had accompanied the Macys on their European tour in 1893. Agnes Carpenter was Everit's sister-in-law, and she and her mother Josephine were also longtime Macy family friends.

[5] The bungalow remained in Alice's family through the 1980s; much of Alice's personal property, as well as items belonging to Kate and Walter, stayed with the family.

[6] KML, p. 73.

[7] *Boston Daily Globe*, June 22, 1915, p. 4.

[8] Ibid.

[9] KML, p. 73 and W. Barry Thomson, "Summary History of the Yacht 'Wenonah' Built 1914-1915 for Walter Graeme Ladd and Kate Macy Ladd," May 2009.

[10] The *Weekly Exponent*, July 22, 1915, was the local Peapack newspaper at that time.

[11] KML, p. 90.

[12] Ibid, p. 76.

[13] Ibid, p. 94.

[14] Ibid, p. 96. The hostess was Madeleine Force Astor, the young widow of John Jacob Astor who perished in the sinking of the *Titanic* in 1912. *The New York Times*, January 19, 1916.

[15] KML, pp. 81-82.

[16] Ibid, p. 79.

[17] Charles W. Burr, M.D. "The S. Weir Mitchell Oration." Delivered before the College of Physicians of Philadelphia, November 19, 1919, and published by the College in 1920. Dr. Burr was one of Mitchell's former students and colleagues. He and Kate became well acquainted during the course of her rest cure in 1892. The Ladds gave a gift of $40,000, almost one million dollars in today's money.

[18] See Lillian Wald, *The House on Henry Street,* (New York: Henry Holt and Co., 1915) and Elizabeth Fee and Liping Bu, "Origins of Public Health Nursing: The Henry Street Visiting Nurse Service," *American Journal of Public Health*, July 2010, 100 (7) pp. 1206-1207.

[19] *Our First One Hundred Years 1904-2004, Visiting Nurse Association of Somerset Hills* (no publication details provided).

[20] Annual Report of the Visiting Nurse Association of Somerset Hills, New Jersey, 1913-1914, pp. 9 and 11.

[21] Minutes of the Raritan River Sub-committee, 12-2-15. Kate wanted to insure safe transport for a new nurse. The previous year a much-loved nurse was killed when the automobile she was driving on her rounds crashed.

[22] Ibid.

[23] Annual Report of Visiting Nurse Association of Somerset Hills, New Jersey, 1916, p. 16.

[24] Minutes of the Raritan River Sub-Committee, March 2, 1916.

[25] KML, p. 89.

[26] Annual Report of the Visiting Nurse Association of Somerset Hills New Jersey, 1916, pp. 17-18.

[27] Ibid.

Chapter 27

[1] KML, pp. 86-87.

[2] *The Berry School News*, March 7, 1917.

[3] Telegraph sent from Bernardsville, NJ, to Rome, GA, on December 1, 1927.

[4] KML, p. 86.

[5] From a letter written by Alice Lemley to Martha M. Berry, March 20, 1915

[6] KML, p. 87.

[7] *The Berry School News*, March 7, 1917.

[8] *Southern Highlander*, Fall-Winter, 1945-46, p. 19.

[9] Ouida Dickey and Doyle Mathis, *Berry College, A History,* (Athens, GA: The University of Georgia Press, 2005), pp. 67-69.

[10] *The Newark Sunday News*, July 2, 1967.

Chapter 28

[1] KML, p. 103.

[2] Ibid, p. 100.

[3] Ibid, pp. 110-111.

[4] Augusta P. Hope to Martha M. Berry, February 21, 1917.

[5] KML, p. 111.

[6] State of New York, Department of Health of the City of New York Bureau of Records Certificate of Death #7099, Alice Lemley, February 24, 1917. Alice's death certificate gave her birth date as January 27, 1869; all other records indicate that she was born in 1870.

[7] KML, pp. 112-113.

[8] Augusta P. Hope to Martha M. Berry, February 26, 1917.

[9] KML, pp. 112-113.

[10] *Daily Local News*, West Chester, Chester County, PA. February 28, 1917.

[11] Augusta P. Hope to Martha M. Berry, February 26, 1917, and Martha M. Berry to Augusta P. Hope, March 2, 1917.

[12] KML, pp. 113-116.

[13] Report of the Raritan River Sub-Committee of the Visiting Nurse Association of Somerset Hills, 1920-1921, p. 28.

Chapter 29
[1] Maple Cottage ledger book, H. Estelle Dudley, 1912.
[2] KML, p. 114.
[3] Ibid, pp. 119-120.
[4] Ibid, p. 123.
[5] Ibid, p. 139.
[6] Ibid.
[7] Ibid, p. 140.
[8] From an interview with Dr. Eric Kast by Robert Mc Cloy as quoted in the *Reader,* a local Chicago publication, September 15, 1983. Eric Kast was a nephew of Ludwig Kast. He stated that his uncle made it possible for him and his parents to leave Europe in 1938. Although they were considered themselves Christians, as Jewish converts to Christianity they feared for their safety under the Nazi regime.
[9] This was the first American institution created to specifically support biomedical research. It was based on the model of the Pasteur Institute in France and the Koch Institute in Germany.
[10] KML, p. 92.
[11] *Musical America,* Vol. 25, 1917, p. 8.

Chapter 30
[1] Christopher Tudico, *The History of the Josiah Macy Foundation,* (New York, NY: Josiah Macy Foundation, 2012), p. 12.
[2] This point is noteworthy as it reflects what is written in Walter's last will and testament, drawn up in February 1932; Kate's will was drawn up at the same time. However, it is also worth noting that although he might have had high regard for Kate's success at Maple Cottage, we find no concrete evidence of his interest or involvement in the convalescent home, leading one to speculate that his 1932 decision about the use of the bulk of his wealth was actually a fulfillment of Kate's wishes.
[3] KML, p. 147.
[4] From a memorandum written by an unidentified Ladd secretary filed with documents pertaining to a Superior Court, Chancery Division investigation regarding the final acceptance of the will of Kate Macy Ladd, Trenton, New Jersey, 1949.
[5] Ibid and "Assignment and Declaration of Trust," Walter G. Ladd to Josiah Macy Jr. Foundation, April 30, 1930, Josiah Macy Jr. Foundation Archives (New York, NY).
[6] KML, p. 236.
[7] Ibid, p. 184.
[8] Ibid, p. 214.
[9] From a memorandum written by an unidentified Ladd secretary, Trenton, New Jersey, 1949.
[10] KML, p. 241.

[11] Ibid, pp. 245-246.

[12] "Assignment and Declaration of Trust," Walter G. Ladd to Josiah Macy Jr. Foundation, April 30, 1930, Josiah Macy Jr. Foundation Archives (New York, NY).

[13] As quoted in *The History of the Josiah Macy Foundation,* Christopher Tudico, (New York: Josiah Macy Jr. Foundation, 2012), p. 13.

[14] Walter was seventy-three when he took possession of the yacht. The agreement through which he received all of Kate's surplus income terminated on December 31, 1929. His last payment was in the amount of $829,501.94. The termination of the agreement was in connection with the organization of Kate's foundation. See records of the Superior Court, Chancery Division, Trenton, New Jersey, re: final accounting of the will of Kate Macy Ladd, 1949.

[15] Phoebe Edgar Testimony, State of New Jersey Department of Taxation and Finance Transfer Inheritance Tax Bureau, 1949, p. 6.

[16] KML, pp. 267-268.

[17] From an unpublished biography by Fred Irwin, 1974, Chapter IV, p. 23 (V. Everit Macy Papers, Westchester County Archives, Elmsford, NY).

[18] KML, p. 268.

[19] *The New York Times,* March 28, 1930.

[20] Phoebe Edgar Testimony, State of New Jersey Department of Taxation, 1949, p. 45.

[21] Kate Macy Ladd Letter of Gift, April 24, 1930, Josiah Macy Jr. Foundation Archives (New York, NY).

[22] *The New York Times*, April 25, 1930, and *New York Evening World*, April 25, 1930.

[23] Michel Anctil, *Te Vega, The Story Of A Schooner And Her People*, (Privately published, 2011), p. 20. *Etak* has enjoyed a much more spectacular reign on the sea than the Ladds' yacht *Wenonah*. The schooner has been meticulously maintained under the flag of several nations; more than one dozen people have owned her since 1933. In 2016, Walter's beloved schooner was on the market again with a new name, *Deva*. Her asking price was $6,500,000 Euros.

[24] Clarence G. Michalis, Forward, *The Josiah Macy Jr. Foundation, 1930-1955: A Review of Activities,* (New York: Josiah Macy Jr. Foundation, 1955), p. 3, as quoted in Christopher Tudico, *The History of the Josiah Macy Jr. Foundation,* (New York: Josiah Macy Jr. Foundation, 2012), p. 23.

[25] Josiah Macy Jr. Foundation, Minutes of the Annual Meeting, October 15, 1930.

[26] This seems like a paltry sum being that it was resolved that the sum of $5,000 was set aside as a reserve for the purchase of office furniture if necessary.

[27] *The New York Times*, October 16, 1930.

[28] *TIME Magazine,* October 27, 1930.

[29] Christopher Tudico, *The History of the Josiah Macy Jr. Foundation,* (New York: Josiah Macy Jr. Foundation, 2012), pp. 21-22. See also www.macyfoundation.org/news/entry/the-macy-story.

[30] Einstein relied heavily on "Walther" Mayer, a fellow Jew whose future in Europe was also in jeopardy. He refused to join the staff of the new Institute for Advanced Studies at Princeton until he was fully certain that a position was being held for Mayer as well. The men and their wives finally immigrated to the United States in 1933 and settled in Princeton, New Jersey. See also Abraham Pais, *Subtle is The Lord, The Science and Life of Albert Einstein*, (New York: Oxford University Press, Inc., 2005), p. 492. The extent to which the Kast-Einstein friendship continued once Einstein was located so close to Natirar is not known.

[31] For further detail about the work of Dr. Helen Flanders Dunbar, see *The Journal of Religion and Health,* Curtis W. Hart, "Helen Flanders Dunbar: Helen Flanders Dunbar: Physician, Medievalist, Enigma," Vol. 35, No. 1, Spring 1996, pp. 50-51.

[32] Since 1939, this publication has been the official peer reviewed organ of the American Psychosomatic Society. In 2018, the society produced Volume 80 of the journal.

[33] Kate Macy Ladd to Ludwig Kast, April 6, 1932, Josiah Macy Jr. Foundation Archives (New York, NY).

Chapter 31

[1] From a conversation with E.Macy Schoenborn, February, 2018.

[2] KML, p. 227.

[3] Interview with S. Fisher, July 6, 2009.

[4] Letter written by Ruby Firlotte to Nicholas Meany, Summer 1929.

[5] *The Bar Harbor Times,* August 27, 1930.

[6] Ibid.

[7] KML, p. 269.

[8] Paul Smart, executor to estate of Walter G. Ladd, 1933.

[9] *TIME Magazine*, "Richest Hospital," February 17, 1930.

[10] *The Bar Harbor Times*, May 24, 1933, and June 7, 1933.

[11] From a letter written by Kate Macy Ladd to Josiah Noel and Polly Macy, August 9, 1933. Adolph Dick was Julia Dick Macy's unmarried brother.

[12] *The New York Sun*, March 11, 1935.

[13] Last will and testament of Walter G. Ladd, February 23, 1932.

[14] Ibid.

Chapter 32

[1] *The New York Times*, December 17, 1935.

[2] Ibid, October 30, 1936, and November 9, 1937.

[3] Christopher Tudico, *The History of the Josiah Macy Jr. Foundation*, p. 30.

[4] Ibid, pp. 31-33.

[5] Hearing Held in the Matter of the Estate of Kate Macy Ladd (November 16, 1949), pp. 35-36, Testimony of Phoebe Edgar.

[6] Ibid, pp. 51-52.

[7] Ibid, p. 22, Testimony of Lawrence Morris.

[8] Affidavit of Dr. Andrew G. Foord, December 14, 1949, from notes provided by W. Barry Thomson.

[9] Hearing Held in the Matter of the Estate of Kate Macy Ladd, (November 16, 1949), p. 4, Testimony of Dr. Willard C. Rappleye.

[10] Ibid, pp. 7.

[11] Ibid, pp. 5-6. Note: The term functional disorder had its origin in the 1920s, the term du jour for what seemed to be a medical condition that remained largely undetected under a physical examination.

[12] Hearing Held in the Matter of the Estate of Kate Macy Ladd (November 16, 1949), p. 21, Testimony of Lawrence Morris.

[13] Ella A. Fletcher, *The Philosophy of Rest*, (New York, NY: Dodge Co., 1906), p. 10.

[14] Ibid, p. 23.

[15] *Autumn Leaves From Maple Cottage*, (Portland, ME, The Mosher Press, 1919), pp. 22-23. Author unattributed.

[16] Hearing Held in the Matter of the Estate of Kate Macy Ladd (November 16, 1949), p. 8, Testimony of Dr. Willard C. Rappleye.

[17] Ibid, p. 68, Testimony of Phyllis Temple Woodruff.

[18] From an undated letter written by Regina O'Hara to a friend who was convalescing at the Kate Macy Ladd Home.

[19] Conversation with E. Macy Schoenborn, Whitemarsh, PA, January 28, 2018. Edith's stepfather was the son of an Italian prince and Jane Allen Campbell who was an American woman from New Jersey.

[20] Ibid.

[21] From an interview with E. Tickner Silver, Pennington, NJ, November 30, 2012.

[22] Ibid.

[23] Ibid.

[24] Hearing Held in the Matter of the Estate of Kate Macy Ladd (November 16, 1949), pp. 71-72, Testimony of Dr. Isaac Ogden Woodruff.

[25] Ibid, pp. 75-78.

[26] Robert Moats Miller, *Harry Emerson Fosdick, Preacher, Pastor, Prophet*, (New York and Oxford; Oxford University Press, 1985), pp. 379-388.

[27] From an interview with E.Tickner Silver, Pennington, NJ, March 21, 2018.

EPILOGUE

[1] Kate Macy Ladd Letter of Gift, April 24, 1930, Josiah Macy Jr. Foundation Archives (New York, N.Y.).

[2] Anne Harrington, *The Cure Within: A History of Mind-Body Medicine*, (New York, NY: W.W. Norton, 2008),V and Kathy Quinn Thomas, "The Mind-Body Connection: Granny Was Right After All." *Rochester Review*, Vol. 59, No. 3, 1997. Available online at www.rochester.edu/pr/Review/V59N3/feature 2.html.

[3] The age requirement for admission varied slightly throughout the Home's history.

[4] As quoted anonymously in the "Five Year Report Kate Macy Ladd Convalescent Home, Far Hills, New Jersey."

[5] *The New York Times,* September 23, 1945.

[6] The Thirty-fourth Annual Report of the Kate Macy Ladd Convalescent Home, Far Hills, NJ, 1982.

[7] *The Bernardsville News*, Vol. 85, No. 43, October 13, 1983, and "History and Closing Report of Kate Macy Ladd Convalescent Home, Far Hills, New Jersey, 1949-1983" prepared by administrator Barry L. Mills and Staff.

[8] *The New York Times*, June 27, 1983.

Made in the USA
Middletown, DE
29 July 2019